SUPERNOVA WOMAN

REIMAGINING YOUR LIFE AFTER 50

MARIANNE CLYDE

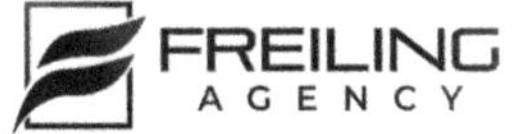

First Paperback and Hardback Editions

Some names, businesses, places, events, locales, incidents, and identifying details inside this book have been changed to protect the privacy of individuals.

Published by Freiling Agency, LLC.

P.O. Box 1264
Warrenton, VA 20188

www.FreilingAgency.com

PB ISBN: 978-1-963701-99-9
HB ISBN: 978-1-963701-09-8
E-book ISBN: 978-1-963701-08-1

Dedication

This book is dedicated to the memory of Susan Starr Allhusen (1948-2024). As her middle name indicates, she was born a star and grew up to be one of the brightest supernovas I have ever had the privilege of having as a friend. Her light has dimmed on this earth but will forever shine in my heart.

Contents

Acknowledgments

Throughout my exploration of stars and supernovas, I have met many fabulous women—some of which are highlighted in this book. They are women of courage, determination, and vision. They don't get caught up in hatred, revenge, or gossip. They know that they are not in competition with anyone. Their goals are varied, but their purpose is the same: to live their lives to the fullest, striving to do the most they can each day to make the world a better place, not looking behind, but looking ahead.

My loving thanks to those who relayed their stories to me to be able to share with you: Jan Molino, Dr. Geeta Mehta, Novita Rumngangun, Dr. Jo Anne Lyon, Susan Allhusen, and Nancy Schulze.

I am grateful to the TEDx Warrenton team that allowed me to hone and share my message, *Descendants of the Stars*: Mike Schmidtmann, Jan Fox, Tara Helkowski, Louis McDonald, Rachel Price, and Tracy Reidel. I also want to thank Daphne Latimore, Lisa Olsen, and others who spoke that day and inspired me.

Thanks also to Tom Freiling and his team at the Freiling Agency for a genuine interest in the success of this book—using a very hands-on approach to ensure that the message gets out to women changemakers everywhere.

And, of course, to Bob Clyde, my partner and biggest supporter, with whom I share this unbelievable adventure that I call my life.

Introduction

Middle age is the time to become the woman you're meant to be!

Once you hit a certain age, you begin to feel your best years are behind you, right?

Indeed, it's common for women to feel like they're expected to coast for the rest of their lives, to just watch the world and their own lives go by. Women often give up when they reach middle age. They hit menopause, get tired, and decide it's too hard to continue to push forward. The changes in their bodies and lives seem overwhelming, leading to a sense of resignation. They feel pressure to conform to a passive role, letting go of dreams, ambitions, and the pursuit of personal growth.

As a therapist and coach, I hear it all the time.

Jennifer, a vibrant and accomplished woman in her early fifties, came to me feeling lost and defeated. She had been a successful professional, a devoted mother, and an active member of her church and community. However, as she entered her fifties, she began to feel the weight of exhaustion and self-doubt. The physical symptoms were challenging enough, but it was the emotional toll that hit her hardest. She felt like she was losing her sense of purpose and identity.

"It's like I've hit a wall," Jennifer said during one of our sessions. "I used to have so much energy and drive, but now I just feel drained. It's hard to keep up with everything, and sometimes I don't know if I can find the strength to push forward. I feel like I'm trapped. I don't even know who I am anymore."

Jennifer's story is not unique. Many women experience a similar sense of stagnation during this period of their lives. Their children are growing up, and now they feel like they're expected to coast for the rest of their lives, to watch the world and their own lives go by. Grab your rocking chair and get out the knitting needles!

For other women, they are not necessarily missing the drive but the execution. They feel like they've missed out, and a giant gap now exists that prevents them from letting go of the pause button. Most men don't pause; they keep going. But for women, the role of being a mom often means putting their own dreams and ambitions on hold. While men are generally encouraged to pursue their goals continuously, women frequently find themselves prioritizing the needs of their families over their own aspirations. This creates a challenging void, especially in terms of creating a new career. This is not a criticism, but it is a fact.

However, middle age doesn't have to be a time of giving up. On the contrary, it's the time to become the woman you're meant to be!

When I spoke about this to a room full of women during my TEDx Talk, I saw heads vigorously nodding in agreement. A few even clapped their hands, expressing their enthusiasm and understanding. It was as if they were saying, "Yes, Marianne, we get it! We've been there, and we feel the same way!" It was reassuring but also discouraging because I knew many women would leave the room and not change a thing.

They would go back to their same lives and not get much further than wishing and hoping that things would get better.

There's a big difference between wishing things would change and making them change. Wishing is passive, a hope that circumstances will improve on their own. Making things change, however, requires action, determination, and a willingness to take control of your own destiny. It's about recognizing that you have the power to influence your life and taking the necessary steps to create the future you want.

That's why I decided to write this book. Women, it's time to stop wishing upon a star and be the star you were created to be. It's time to be a Supernova woman!

This stage of life can be a time of incredible transformation and empowerment. It's a period where you have the opportunity to redefine yourself, to embrace the wisdom and experience you've gained, and to take control of your future with renewed vigor. Rather than succumbing to the expectation of slowing down, you can choose to see this as a new beginning. It's time to speed up!

This book is about taking that control, about breaking free from the stereotypes and limitations that society places on middle-aged women. It's about finding the courage to continue pushing forward, to keep striving for what you want, and to live a life filled with purpose and joy. It's about disrupting your life and the lives of everyone around you, maybe even around the world.

Disruption is how we change the world; doing what others can't or won't do. Disruption is not as difficult or offensive as you might think. It's pretty much just following your own truth, unapologetically. That's what I teach women to do, and it's what I want to share with you in this book. I'm going to reveal to you my own journey of disruption, from the serene summit of Mt. Fuji, to the heart-pounding excitement of freefalling from 10,000 feet out of an airplane, to the peace and serenity of becoming a star-watcher.

Along the way, I've learned invaluable lessons about the power of resilience, determination, and self-belief. Join me as we explore how you too can unlock your inner adventurer and live a life filled with passion, purpose, and pride. This is your moment to step boldly into the unknown and embrace the adventure that lies ahead. Whether it's running your first marathon (I did it, you can too!), publishing a best-selling book, traveling the world helping women in poverty, or starting your own business, every journey begins with a single step. In fact, you've already taken the first step by opening up this book!

Doesn't it already feel good to know that you're not alone in this journey?

I'm here to remind you that many women have faced the same challenges and have emerged stronger and more fulfilled. By sharing their stories, insights, and practical advice, this book aims to inspire and empower you to take charge of your life. It's never too late to start anew, to pursue your dreams, and to create a future that excites and motivates you. So, let's embark on this journey together. Let's redefine what it means to be a middle-aged woman. Let's take control of our futures and show the world that our best years are not behind us, but ahead of us. The power to shape your destiny is within you, and this book is here to guide you every step of the way.

Take a deep breath, summon your courage, and let's become Supernova women together.

I'm chomping at the bit to share with you the deep, age-old wisdom that I've learned along the way so you can grasp the vision and fly with me to heights you've never thought possible!

CHAPTER 1

The Supernova Woman

Like the supernova, this is not an end but a new beginning, filled with brilliant stars.

"What's a Supernova woman, Marianne?" This question is posed to me by women every day, from all corners of the globe. I'm incredibly grateful for their curiosity, and I never tire of explaining my fascination with the similarities between a star in crisis and a woman experiencing menopause. Admittedly, I might be the first to make this unique connection! Allow me to explain.

You might say I'm an amateur astronomer. After my children were mostly grown, I traveled to Sierra Leone, West Africa, to work with men, women, and children affected by war. It was an emotional time for me, both because of my own life transitions and because I'm an empathic person. The pain and suffering around me were almost too much to bear, leaving a deep impression on my heart.

One night, while taking a long walk and reflecting, I looked up at the dark night sky. With minimal light pollution and vast, open spaces, stargazing in Africa offers some of the most remarkable opportunities on Earth. I stared at the sky for quite a while that night and picked out the Orion constellation, located on the celestial equator. It's one of the brightest constellations, so it's not hard to find. I found comfort in its constancy and returned each night. I learned stargazing has a peaceful, meditative effect on the soul. Focusing on the stars can quiet your mind, reduce stress, and promote relaxation. This mindfulness can lead to a greater sense of well-being.

But stargazing also connects you to something vast and timeless. The stars have been shining for billions of years, seen by countless generations. This continuity can be comforting, reminding you that you are part of a larger, enduring universe. And when you look at the immense scale of the cosmos, your daily worries and stresses can seem small and insignificant by comparison. This shift in perspective can help you feel less burdened by the challenges you face, making them easier to manage. Realizing how small you are in the grand scheme of the universe can foster a sense of humility and gratitude. This awareness can help you appreciate the beauty and fragility of life.

So, Orion became a familiar presence in my life. It was inspiring to me. More recently, I also learned about Betelgeuse, the star marking Orion's right shoulder. The name reminded me of the movie "Beetlejuice," making it easier to remember. I discovered that Betelgeuse was beginning to fade and dim, alerting scientists that it was destined to become a *supernova*. This transformation could happen in our lifetime or many years from now, but either way, it means that the star will shine incredibly brightly for about 100,000 years before fading completely.

Frankly, I didn't know much about supernovae, so I'll assume you don't either. In a lay person's words, it basically goes like this:

When a star begins to run out of fuel, its core undergoes significant changes. The star's primary fuel source, hydrogen, starts to deplete after millions or even billions of years of nuclear fusion. As the hydrogen fuel runs out, the star can no longer sustain the nuclear fusion reactions that generate the pressure needed to counteract the force of gravity. At this critical juncture, the star's core collapses under the immense force of gravity. This rapid collapse generates temperatures and pressures so extreme that the core implodes, creating a shockwave that causes the outer layers of the star to explode outward in a spectacular event known as a supernova. It's a process of stellar death and rebirth and is a vital part of the cosmic cycle, contributing to the ongoing evolution of the universe.

When a star undergoes this transformation, it doesn't just end in destruction; it also marks the beginning of new possibilities and formations.

Does that sound familiar to you? I thought so! The pull of gravity usually gets a few chuckles (and tears!) when I compare a woman in menopause to the stars! What's happening to my body!? What's happening to my life!?

Like a supernova, women going through menopause experience profound changes as her body transitions out of its reproductive phase. The primary fuel source for a woman's reproductive system—her hormones—begins to deplete after decades of menstruation and fertility. As hormone levels decline, the body can no longer sustain the reproductive processes that have been in place for so long. This critical juncture brings about significant physical and emotional changes, akin to the collapse of a star's core.

But I'm not a doctor and I'm not referring simply to a woman's biological response to hormones. When a woman turns around age 50, life itself begins to change. Everything and everyone around them begin to look and feel different. Many women feel like they are imploding. They feel like their star is dimming. My mission is to remind women that this time of life can mark the beginning of new possibilities and formations. It's time to shine more brightly. Like the supernova, this is not just an end but a new beginning, filled with potential for brilliant moments ahead.

Yes, I believe it's time for you to shine your brightest! This is my message to women as I write, travel and speak, and coach women who are trying to reimagine their lives. Your star is not dying. On the contrary, it's exploding with new life.

Will you be a supernova? Keep reading, keep moving, keep telling yourself that this is your time!

CHAPTER 2

What to Expect

Unless you specially name how you want to feel, you will stay where you are: unhappy.

You don't have to love where you are in life. You may hate it. But you do have to accept it.

You may find yourself in a difficult or complicated situation such as being unexpectedly fired from a job or going through the emotional and logistical challenges of a divorce. You might not like where you live. You might be bored out of your mind. You might be overweight or unhealthy.

Whether these events were by choice or circumstances outside your control, they are real and they are happening to you. They are your reality.

It's natural to feel a strong urge to deny these painful realities, to shake your head and insist, "This is not happening to me." However, such denial only serves to keep you stagnant, unable to move forward or address the situation constructively. If you refuse to admit your feelings or you nurture negative emotions like anger, bitterness, unforgiveness, hatred, guilt, or shame, you are removing the power that you have within you to change. Embracing the reality of your difficult thoughts and moments is crucial for your growth and recovery.

The first step is acknowledging the situation without judgment. Recognize that it's okay to feel upset or confused; these are normal reactions. Go ahead, say it:

I'm angry.
I'm bored.
I don't like my job.
I'm sick.
I'm poor.
I don't like being in debt.
I'm jobless.
I'm lonely.
I don't like my marriage.
I'm tired.
I'm frustrated.
I don't like my house.
I'm anxious.
I'm overwhelmed.
I don't like the weather here.
I'm sad.
I'm scared.

Then, begin to consider how you want to feel. You don't need a plan yet. Just proclaim to yourself how you'd rather be. Unless you specially name how you want to feel, you will stay where you are: unhappy. Let me make it simple: If you don't like spicy food, but you don't acknowledge it and keep on going to a Mexican restaurant, you aren't going to be happy with dinner! Yes, it's really that simple.

So, once you've told yourself what you don't want and like, and what you'd prefer, then (and only then) will you be able to change things. You can stop eating Mexican food.

Finally, you can then take practical steps towards adaptation and resilience. This might involve seeking support from friends, family, or professionals such as counselors, who can provide guidance and perspective during this challenging time. It might also mean planning strategically for the next phases of your life, whether that's updating your resume and exploring new career opportunities, or understanding your legal rights and responsibilities in a divorce.

By facing the situation head-on and actively engaging with the necessary steps to navigate through it, you not only regain a sense of control but also open the door to new possibilities and beginnings. Remember you can't control other people. You can't control a lot of the things that happen to you. But you can control your response. And you can plan to change those things you can control.

Women often fall into a trap of accepting too much. We over-accept. In many cases, this over-acceptance comes at a high personal cost. Supernova women run straight at this problem. We readily acknowledge what we don't like about ourselves and our situation. Then we aim to change it and accept those things we simply cannot change.

CHAPTER 3

New Habits for a New You

Cumulative sustained efforts result in habits.
And habits result in a new YOU.

So, you've crafted a dream and laid out a detailed plan to achieve it. What comes next is perhaps THE most crucial step: putting that plan into action!

Now it's time to roll up your sleeves and get to work. The key ingredient that will turn your plan into reality is your commitment to consistently executing it, day after day. If you don't work on it most days, you will end up working on it less and less until you eventually give-up. I've seen so many women give-up, which is disheartening. Don't be THAT one! Force yourself to be consistent.

Success doesn't come from sporadic bursts of effort but from the steady, ongoing application of your skills and strategies. This means dedicating yourself to working on your goals at least most days, even when motivation wanes or obstacles arise. That's the tough part because on some days, this might mean taking huge strides forward; while on others, it might simply be about maintaining momentum with smaller, more manageable tasks.

What's important is the cumulative effect of this sustained effort over time. Cumulative sustained efforts result in habits. And habits result in a new YOU!

Developing new habits is essential for transforming your dreams into achievable goals. Start by breaking down your larger goals into small, manageable tasks that can be tackled daily. For instance, if your goal is to write a book, set a habit of writing a specific number of words each day. Make these tasks part of your routine by scheduling them at consistent times, which helps solidify them into habits. Tools such as planners, apps, or reminders can assist in keeping you accountable. Don't make the mistake of thinking you can keep it all in your head (been there, done that!).

Furthermore, it's so important to cultivate an environment that supports your new habits. An environment tailored to your goals can enhance focus, increase productivity, and make it easier to maintain the discipline needed to stick to your new habits. When your space is organized and aligned with your objectives, it reduces the likelihood of distractions and unnecessary stress, which can derail your progress. For example, if your goal is to exercise regularly, having a dedicated space at home with your workout equipment readily accessible can encourage you to engage in physical activity more consistently. Similarly, if you're aiming to study or write, a quiet, clutter-free area can promote mental clarity and concentration.

Moreover, an environment that reflects your commitments can reinforce your identity as someone who lives by their goals. It becomes a physical manifestation of your dedication and serves as a constant reminder of what you're striving to achieve. This supportive setting not only facilitates the practical aspects of forming new habits but also psychologically embeds these habits into your daily life, making them easier to sustain.

Creating a supportive setting might mean displaying flowers, or organizing your workspace to encourage productivity, or perhaps it involves limiting distractions during your designated work times. Also, consider finding a community or a partner who shares similar goals. This community can provide both motivation and accountability. As these daily actions become more routine, they lose their sense of effort and transform into automatic behaviors that steadily drive you towards your ultimate objectives.

Remember, the power of habit lies in repetition and consistency, so stay committed and watch as small daily actions accumulate into substantial achievements.

This commitment also involves continuously refining your approach based on feedback and results. Be adaptive and willing to adjust your strategies as necessary. Remember, persistence doesn't mean doing the same thing repeatedly if it's not working; it means being committed enough to your goal to adapt your methods until you find success. In summation, the transition from dream to reality is bridged by the commitment to consistently work towards your goal, making smart adjustments along the way.

Finally, I'm a big believer in CELEBRATING your successes. When you reach a milestone, treat yourself. Remember you are the creator of your life. Maintaining positive energy is important, so learn to pay attention to how you are feeling!

CHAPTER 4

Hit the Reset Button

The real magic happens when you break those aspirations into actionable steps.

Women often find themselves so deeply entrenched in the roles they've always known as mothers, partners, and working professionals, somewhere along the way they forget to set new goals for themselves. The inertia of routine sets in, and before they realize it, they're stuck in a rut, wondering where their dreams and ambitions disappeared.

But here's the thing: life isn't static, and neither should your goals be. Just because you've reached a certain age doesn't mean your journey is over. In fact, it's quite the opposite! Now is the time to reimagine your life. This can be a time for profound growth, but only if you're willing to embrace the change and set new goals for yourself.

So, if you find yourself feeling stagnant, it's time to hit the reset button. Take a moment to reflect on what truly lights you up inside, what makes you excited to jump out of bed in the morning. Whether it's reigniting an old passion, pursuing a new hobby, or setting ambitious career goals, now is the perfect time to dream big and take action.

Here's the thing about goals though: You've got to break them down. It's not enough to simply cast new visions. Setting goals is just the first step; the real magic happens when you break those aspirations into actionable steps. Think of it like building a house – you can't just envision the final structure; you need blueprints, materials, and a solid foundation. Similarly, breaking your goals into manageable tasks not only makes them less daunting but also increases the likelihood of success.

Accordingly, take the time to outline the specific actions you need to take to reach your objectives. Whether it's daily habits, weekly milestones, or monthly targets, each small step brings you closer to your ultimate goal. Remember, progress is not always linear, and setbacks are a natural part of the journey. What matters most is your resilience and commitment to keep moving forward, one step at a time.

Consider setting goals with actionable objectives in the following areas:

Health: For middle-aged women, health goals often revolve around weight management and fitness, typically entailing exercise and nutrition improvements. Additionally, health goals may involve targeting specific illnesses or diseases for prevention or symptom reduction.

Intellectual: Intellectual goals focus on cognitive growth and learning. This could include pursuing further education, developing new skills, or engaging in intellectual hobbies that stimulate the mind and expand knowledge. Or reading more books!

Relationships: Relationship goals encompass fostering and nurturing meaningful connections with family, friends, romantic partners, and colleagues.

This may involve improving communication, deepening emotional intimacy, and resolving conflicts to cultivate healthier and more fulfilling relationships.

Career: Career goals pertain to professional advancement, skill development, and overall satisfaction in one's work life. This could involve starting your own business or organization, acquiring new certifications, or exploring career changes that align with personal passions and values.

Spiritual: Spiritual goals involve cultivating a sense of purpose, connection, and inner peace. This may include practices such as meditation, prayer, reading the Bible or another spiritual book, mindfulness, or exploring one's beliefs and values to foster spiritual growth and fulfillment.

Financial: Financial goals center around managing money effectively to achieve financial stability, security, and independence. This could involve setting targets for savings, debt reduction, investment planning, and creating a budget to support long-term financial well-being.

Some of the advice I offer may seem self-explanatory, yet I'm consistently struck by the number of women I encounter who haven't broken their goals down into actionable steps. It's natural to indulge in your dreams, but without a concrete plan to transform those dreams into reality, they'll remain a distant fantasy. Dreaming is the initial spark, the ignition of possibility, but the true magic lies in the strategic execution that turns those dreams into tangible achievements! It's the difference between gazing at the stars and charting a course to reach them.

CHAPTER 5

Learning to Dream Again

Rediscovering your dreams is a deeply personal process that doesn't have to be rushed.

There comes a time in every woman's life where she begins to wonder what she wants, and that time is usually when her children leave for college or leave the home.

In the hustle of daily life as a mom, it's remarkably easy to lose touch with your own aspirations. You might even find that it has been years since you last considered what your personal dreams might be. This disconnection from your desires can be disheartening and unsettling, particularly when confronted with the simple yet profound question: "What is it you want?" If you find yourself shaking your head or shrugging your shoulders in response, know that you are not alone in this experience.

Do you feel like you've drifted away from your dreams, often placing the needs and goals of others ahead of their own? This can lead to a sense of having lost a part of oneself over time.

I'm here to tell you that it's not your fault. It's essential to recognize that if you struggle to remember your dreams or if you find yourself without a clear goal, it is not a reflection of any personal failure. All of your external voices and experiences are simply so overpowering that they drown out your inner desires. They make you feel like your dreams are either unrealistic or unimportant.

The good news, however, is that it's never too late to reconnect with what you want and to begin crafting a life that aligns more closely with those desires.

Be patient with yourself.

The first step in this journey is to give yourself permission to dream again. Allow yourself the space and time to explore your interests and passions, no matter how impractical or far-fetched they might seem. Start small by identifying things you enjoy and gradually build upon these interests. Whether it's picking up an old hobby, exploring new career possibilities, or simply trying out new experiences, each small step is a move towards rediscovering your desires.

Moreover, it's crucial to cultivate an environment that supports your self-discovery. This might involve setting boundaries, seeking out supportive communities, or finding mentors who encourage your growth. As you delve deeper into understanding your own wants and needs, you'll likely find clarity and confidence in articulating them to others. This takes time, and time is your friend, not your enemy.

Remember, rediscovering your dreams is a deeply personal process that doesn't have to be rushed. It's about learning to listen to yourself again and valuing your own happiness and fulfillment as much as you do others'. Through this process, you can reclaim the dreams that resonate with your true self, bringing more purpose and joy into your life. You spent the last 10, 20, 30 years getting to where you are now. You aren't going to discover your new self overnight. But that doesn't mean you won't!

If you're having trouble finding the new you, I recommend two strategies. They may seem to work against each other upon first glance, but I firmly believe you need to do both.

First, work on the internal you. This process often begins with introspection, where you might engage in activities like journaling, meditation, or therapy to better understand your emotional landscape and thought patterns. It's about questioning long-held beliefs and the roles assigned by society to determine if they truly resonate with what you genuinely feel and want. As this journey unfolds, moments of self-discovery can lead to significant insights about your desires, strengths, weaknesses, and purpose, painting a clearer picture of who you are and what you want from life.

Second, work on the external you. This means getting out and engaging with the world in ways that enrich and challenge you. Start by exploring new environments and activities that spark your interest or curiosity. Whether it's taking up a new hobby, traveling to unfamiliar places, attending workshops or seminars in areas you wish to learn more about, or simply changing your routine to include new experiences, each step you take into the unknown helps build a more dynamic and well-rounded self.

Working on the internal you won't help if you don't take the next step of working on the external you, and visa-versa. Do both, have fun, and be patient. Change will happen!

Remember, we're a tribe. Don't hesitate to reach out to other women for help. They want to help. I want to help! We're Supernova women!

CHAPTER 6

Stop Saying You're Sorry

There's absolutely no need to apologize for being yourself.

I always say when you need help with a problem, go find someone who's already solved the problem. That's why I love Jan Molino. Jan is a popular writer, board coach, and CEO of Aspire-Ascend, a consulting firm that specializes in providing a comprehensive portfolio of board and leadership development services to enhance the success of women in leadership positions. She's passionate about women in leadership!

Having spent years advising women about how they can break through the leadership ranks in corporate America, Jan finds certain patterns of behavior which tend to hold women back. She's discovered where many women get stuck: They aren't assertive enough.

Women frequently find themselves at a disadvantage during discussions at the conference table, often conceding ground or yielding to more assertive colleagues. This tendency can undermine their authority and presence in crucial business settings. Additionally, women have a habit of apologizing excessively, which can inadvertently convey a lack of confidence in their decisions and actions.

Would you agree? I thought so!

These patterns not only affect how women are perceived in the workplace but also limit their opportunities for leadership roles and professional advancement.

Mara arrived early to the conference room, her notes neatly organized and her laptop open to the presentation she'd prepared meticulously. As colleagues trickled in, the hum of conversation filled the space.

Tom sauntered in just as Lisa called the meeting to order. "Alright, team," Lisa began, "Let's dive into the quarterly project updates. Mara, you're first."

Mara stood; her hands, slightly trembling. "Thank you, Lisa. Today, I'll overview the progress on our digital transformation initiative."

As Mara began detailing the project milestones, she felt confident, her months of hard work distilled into clear, concise slides. However, when she reached the challenges section, Tom interrupted. "I think we're overlooking a major flaw here," he said, leaning forward, his voice confident and loud.

Mara hesitated; her mouth, dry. "Well, I'm sorry, maybe I missed...," her voice trailed off.

Tom interjected, "I think my approach might more effectively address our resource allocation issues."

Mara nodded, stepping back slightly. "Of course, Tom. Let's hear your thoughts."

The room's attention shifted as Tom detailed his strategy, full of assertive assurances. Mara's initial points were soon overshadowed. She tried to interject a few times, her voice softer, starting each attempt with, "Sorry, if I may..."

Tom continued to dominate the meeting, while Mara politely nodded her head. By the time the meeting ended, the room agreed with Tom, yet if given the opportunity, Mara had already come to the same conclusions.

I'll bet this dialogue makes you angry, right? You're angry Mara didn't speak up. You're mad that she got taken advantage of. Guess what? You are Mara! It's a startling realization, but often, we are more like Mara than we'd like to admit. We've all had moments where we've held back our true thoughts, overly apologized, and allowed others to steer the discourse. Recognizing this is the first step towards making a change in how we communicate and assert ourselves in professional environments.

While there are certainly many ways women can work on and improve their communication skills, you can start by not always apologizing.

Apologizing, when used excessively, and even not excessively, can unintentionally convey a lack of confidence or assertiveness. Instead, focus on expressing ideas and opinions clearly and confidently without prefacing them with an apology unless absolutely necessary. This shift not only strengthens one's communication but also helps in projecting more self-assuredness and authority. By making this adjustment, women can start to change the dynamics of their interactions, ensuring their voices are heard and respected on equal footing with their colleagues.

This habit can be challenging to overcome, but it's crucial. Many women often find themselves apologizing unnecessarily, but there's absolutely no need to apologize for being yourself. This behavior is often the result of societal conditioning that tells women not to attract attention, not to stand out too much, and not to be too confident. Nonsense. Making waves is how you impact the world. Remember, whatever you say or do creates ripples, so why not make them positive?

Here are a few ways you can apologize without apologizing:

Acknowledgment and Appreciation: "Thank you for your patience" or "I appreciate your understanding." This recognizes the situation without directly apologizing.

Offering a Solution: Instead of focusing on the apology, you can say, "Let's see how we can fix this." This shifts the focus from the problem to the solution.

Expressing Empathy: "I can see how that might be frustrating." This shows that you are empathetic towards the other person's feelings without admitting fault.

Affirming Action: "I'll make sure this is handled right away." This indicates that you are taking responsibility for resolving any issues without dwelling on the mistake.

Requesting Feedback: "How can we improve this to meet your expectations?" This involves the other person in finding a resolution and moves the conversation forward positively.

The next time you feel the urge to apologize, take a moment to pause before you act. Reflect on the situation: Is there truly a need for an apology, or are you simply defaulting to a habitual response? This pause can give you the opportunity to assess whether your intended apology is necessary or if there might be a more empowering way to address the situation. By stopping to consider your actions, you encourage a more deliberate and confident approach in your interactions.

CHAPTER 7

Find New Energy

You can't control anyone else's mood or state of mind, but you can always control your own.

Have you ever found yourself in a place where the energy seemed palpably negative? Not in a supernatural sense, but rather in the atmosphere of the space, the collective aura of the people present, and the overall ambiance? It's like stepping into a room and instantly feeling a heavy, oppressive atmosphere weighing down on you or encountering a group of individuals whose combined energies create a tense and uncomfortable vibe.

I walked into a meeting once where I could immediately feel the tension. Even before a single word was uttered, the weight of unresolved conflicts and unspoken grievances hung heavily in the air. Despite the veneer of professionalism that attempted to mask the underlying tension, it was impossible to ignore the unease that permeated the room. Every glance exchanged, every hesitant pause in conversation, served as a stark reminder of the simmering discord lurking just beneath the surface.

Been there, done that, right? That's what I mean about bad energy.

The fact is, we all emit energy all the time. Our thoughts inform our feelings which inform our words and actions. If you're happy, you give off happy energy, which permeates the people around you. Conversely, if you're angry, it shows and it can trigger the people around you. We all know this about ourselves and others, yet we often forget how much it impacts our lives.

If you pay attention to how you feel around certain people or in certain places or in certain situations, you'll begin to become more aware of how our surroundings affect us and how we affect our surroundings. Armed with this tiny bit of knowledge, you will be able to see that the air around us also creates ripples when we move, think, act, and speak. You are influencing people around you, based on your mood, all the time.

Without getting too mystical, I think it's really important to recognize the tangible impact our internal processes have on our external experiences. David R. Hawkins, world famous author and researcher on consciousness, identified 17 levels of "consciousness" from high to low, or positive energy to negative energy:

Enlightenment
Peace
Joy
Love
Reason
Acceptance
Willingness
Neutrality
Courage
Pride
Anger
Desire
Fear

Grief
Apathy
Guilt
Shame

In essence, Hawkins emphasizes the importance of aligning with positive energy and states of consciousness as a pathway to personal growth, spiritual evolution, and the realization of one's highest potential. Through practices such as mindfulness, self-awareness, and intentional living, individuals can cultivate a greater sense of inner peace, harmony, and connection with the universal energy that permeates all of existence.

While that might seem a bit too esoteric, it's pragmatically true that angry people are difficult to be around. Joyful, happy, purposeful people inspire you to do better. Sad, depressed people can pull you down emotionally. Positive, inspiring people can lift you up. When you are completely conscious of the kinds of energy you surround yourself with and pick up from others, you can begin to control what kind of energy you put out. You certainly can't control anyone else's mood or state of mind, but you can always control your own. And you can train yourself to get better and more purposeful at it.

People either operate from an internal locus of control or an external locus of control.

If you are operating from your inner strength, knowing that you have power within you to create the life you want by your choices, you become conscious about every decision you make. Those decisions can make a difference in direction which brings strength, creating a purposeful way of living. We understand that we control our mindset and feelings and can influence our attitude from within.

On the other hand, an external locus of control, implies that outside influences like circumstances, other people, and natural disasters are in control of your life, exerting power on the individual so that we then become victims.

I think of heavy energy as weighing us down and light energy as lifting us up. If I allow myself to be overcome by negative energy, I cannot build a positive, powerful life. So, in order to direct my life the way I want it, I have to focus on cultivating lighter, more positive energies like love and joy and peace. These generate a force in my life that overcomes obstacles, breaks through opposition, and builds an inspiring and beautiful future not only for myself but for those who come after me.

It took me a long time to recognize the effects of positive or negative energy in myself and in others around me; but by being attuned to it, I eventually gained more control over my own emotions, my words, and my actions.

This recognition is how we can begin to raise the positive energy on the planet! Will you join me?

CHAPTER 8

Take the First Step

The women I know who are thriving do not allow themselves to be isolated.

Geeta Mehta is a friend and mentor, an award-winning Supernova woman, who built a global network and non-profit organization to help fund micro banks and village knowledge centers in Asia. She is the founder of Asia Initiatives, an organization that works with under-served communities to help transform their neighborhoods through advocacy and improvement of public spaces and homes. Much of their work is done by local groups of women, identifying issues that need to be addressed such as child marriage and education, while creating solutions that are workable and effective in their communities.

A professor at Columbia University and a skilled urban designer, Geeta has garnered attention for her urban design projects in numerous countries including India, China, Ukraine, Brazil, Jamaica, and Ghana. She's my "poster child" for how I love to see women build and thrive in community with each other.

I talk a lot about communities and why women should pay close attention to them. The women I know who are thriving, all share a common trait: They do not allow themselves to be isolated. They actively seek out and engage with other women, understanding the impact these networks can have on their overall well-being and success. It's not always easy, but it's easier than doing nothing.

What happens when you do nothing? If you don't build or find a new community, it often leads to feelings of loneliness, depression, and a sense of disconnection from the world around you. Women are inherently social creatures, who thrive on interaction and shared experiences—even if you think of yourself as an introvert, like I do. But by prioritizing community involvement, you can create a new robust support system that offers emotional and practical assistance during life's challenges.

Here's what happens to many women around age 50:

The transition of children leaving home is often a troubling and confusing turning point for a woman, impacting her friendships and sense of existing community. Often, a younger woman's social circle and daily interactions revolve around her children's activities, school events, and parenting groups. As these connections naturally diminish, women find that many of their established relationships wither away.

Sometimes this transition can happen rather suddenly. You wake up one morning expecting to organize a playdate, grab coffee with a mom group, or attend a school event, only to realize that those familiar routines and social interactions have abruptly ceased. The children have moved out, and the daily bustle that once dictated your schedule has vanished. Poof! Now you're alone!

But you don't have to stay alone. Again, I know it's never easy to walk out the door and go find a new group of "you's." I want to encourage you to embrace the power within you to transform your life by stepping out and finding new relationships and communities. Life is an incredible journey filled with opportunities for growth, connection, and joy, and it begins the moment you decide to engage with the world around you. You have so much to offer and so much to gain from others. By actively seeking out new friendships and becoming part of vibrant communities, you open yourself up to a wealth of experiences, support, and inspiration.

I, a self-proclaimed introvert, make it a point to meet women, old and new friends, for lunch or coffee every week. I also actively seek to align with networking groups that help me stay sharp in my business and in my personal life. These groups not only support me in achieving my goals, they also give me opportunities to share what I can contribute to help others.

Don't let fear or doubt hold you back. Take that first step, attend that event, join that group, and reach out to others. You deserve to live a life filled with meaningful connections and endless possibilities. Your new tribe is out there, waiting to welcome you with open arms. Go out and find them, and watch as your world expands in beautiful, unexpected ways.

It might not be a global network like my friend Geeta has built. In fact, it might be just a small group of new friends, experiencing new things and making a new impact. Large or small, in your neighborhood or across the seas, it matters not how many or where. What matters is that you don't withdraw. It's not time to feel sorry for yourself. You're amazing! It's time to let that amazing woman out of herself and make something happen!

CHAPTER 9

Find a New Way to Make a Difference

Purpose can be found in the simple yet profound act of showing up for others in their time of need.

In the wake of tragedy in Jakarta, Indonesia, Novita Rumngangun's presence gave hope to a young mother grappling with the death of her husband. While loving friends and neighbors offering condolences surrounded the widow, Novita arrived bearing not just sympathy, but practical assistance in the form of an insurance claim check.

As the young mother spoke, her voice quivered with a mixture of gratitude and sorrow. "Many friends come by," she began, her words punctuated by pauses as if each syllable carried the weight of her grief, "and speak of their sympathy and sorrow." She paused, her eyes meeting Novita's with a raw intensity. "I appreciate that so much," she continued, her voice breaking slightly, "but they all go home and live their lives. With this check, you have given my baby and me the ability to continue to live our lives."

The weight of the young mother's words hung heavily in the air. Novita stood frozen, her heart pounding in her chest as she absorbed the gravity of the moment. In that instant, everything seemed to crystallize around her—the pain, the loss, the resilience of the human spirit.

Tears welled in Novita's eyes as she realized the profound impact of her actions. This was more than just a transaction; it was a lifeline, a glimmer of hope amidst the darkness. In delivering her first death benefit, Novita had found her purpose—a calling that transcended the mundane routines of everyday life.

As she stood there, Novita knew with unwavering certainty that she was exactly where she was meant to be. This was her moment, her awakening to the power of compassion and empathy. And in that moment, she made a silent vow to honor the trust placed in her, to be a beacon of hope for those in need, and to never lose sight of the impact a single act could have on a person's life.

Reflecting on her journey, Novita shared with me her childhood dream of becoming a diplomat, an ambassador for her beloved Indonesia. Now, as the VP Director and GM Agency of Manulife, she sees her role as a way to promote and encourage her predominantly female team of agents. With a mantra that dreams should be big enough to inspire fear, Novita embodies the ethos of striving for excellence at every level.

Despite facing doubts and challenges along the way, Novita embraces each opportunity with determination and resilience. Managing a team of 14,000 people across Indonesia, she draws on her empathy and firsthand experience to connect with and empower her colleagues. Her willingness to share her failures fosters trust and authenticity, qualities she believes are rare but invaluable.

For Novita, ambition is not a dirty word; it's a driving force for personal and collective growth. She believes that every woman has a purpose and that aligning one's actions with that purpose brings true fulfillment. As she continues to pursue her goal of being beneficial to others, Novita's journey serves as an inspiration to Supernovas—individuals striving to make a positive impact on the world, regardless of geographical boundaries.

"It makes me excited every single morning," Novita shared, her eyes bright with purpose. "Ever since I was a little girl, I wanted to be a diplomat, an ambassador for my country. And now, helping people live their lives, I see the importance of it right here. I was a nobody, but I had a big dream!" she recalled with a laugh. "My mom said, 'Then be a superstar. Climb the ladder, all the way to the top!"

Navigating her ascent, Novita encountered doubts and challenges but embraced each one with determination. "I don't know if I can do this!" she admitted to herself when faced with her current position. "But I love the challenge of proving those who underestimate me, wrong."

Her journey, fueled by a belief in purpose and authenticity, resonates deeply. "Every woman has a purpose," Novita reflected, "If you are working toward your goal, according to that purpose, you can be happy."

Novita's story transcends borders, resonating with women striving to make a difference wherever they are. As she continues to inspire and uplift, her legacy shines brightly, a testament to the power of resilience and determination in the face of adversity. She also serves as a poignant reminder that purpose can often be found in the most unexpected places, even in something as seemingly mundane as an insurance check.

In that single moment of despair, Novita's practical assistance not only provided financial support but also offered a glimmer of hope and reassurance to the bereaved mother and her child. It's a testament to the profound impact that acts of kindness and compassion can have on others, highlighting the transformative power of empathy and action. It reminds women everywhere that purpose is not always grandiose or earth-shattering; it can be found in the simple yet profound act of showing up for others in their time of need. As Novita discovered, true fulfillment often lies in the ability to make a difference, no matter how small, in the lives of those around us.

CHAPTER 10

Be Good to Yourself

Giving is important, but so is self-preservation. You matter most.

It's almost as if from the moment we're born, women are handed an invisible rulebook that says, "Your needs come last, darling." Sadly, we've been conditioned to be self-sacrificing superheroes. And it's been going on for thousands of years.

Whether it's the relentless demands of caretaking roles, the expectations of perfection in both personal and professional spheres, or the subtle pressure to prioritize the comfort and happiness of others above her own, this unspoken rulebook weaves its threads through every aspect of a woman's life. It's a silent yet powerful force shaping our attitudes, behaviors, and decisions.

We've been told to:

- Wait our turns.
- Not speak up for ourselves, at least not too loudly.
- Put others' needs before our own, even at the expense of our well-being.
- Sacrifice our ambitions and desires for the sake of familial or societal expectations.
- Suppress our emotions, lest they be perceived as weakness or inconvenience.
- Strive for perfection in every aspect of our lives, from appearance to achievements, often at the cost of our mental and physical health.

- Take on the bulk of household and caregiving responsibilities, regardless of other commitments or aspirations.
- Accept limitations and constraints imposed by gender norms and stereotypes, limiting our potential for growth and fulfillment.
- Navigate a world where our worth is often measured by our ability to conform to traditional gender roles, rather than our individual talents, skills, and aspirations.

While there's nothing wrong with being a giver and placing others' needs before our own, somewhere along the way, we forgot that our own needs are just as important. In the noble pursuit of caring for everyone around us, we inadvertently neglected the vital task of tending to our own well-being. Giving is important, but so is self-preservation. I'm here to tell you that the things you are passionate about matter too.

You matter most. Does that sound selfish? Because it isn't.

Acknowledging your own worth and prioritizing your needs doesn't stem from selfishness; rather, it's an act of self-respect. By recognizing that you matter, that your well-being holds significance, you empower yourself to lead a life of greater fulfillment and joy. Yes, joy! You're allowed to be happy because you are amazing!

Embracing this truth isn't about disregarding the needs of others or adopting an egocentric mindset; instead, it's about fostering a healthy balance between giving and receiving, between nurturing others and nurturing ourselves. It's about reclaiming agency over our lives, asserting our right to pursue happiness and fulfillment unapologetically. So, no, it's not selfish—it's an act of radical self-love and empowerment.

As a counselor and coach, I've sat with many women who tell me they're lonely, despite having spent a lifetime serving other people. It's a paradoxical reality that often goes unnoticed by those around them—their days filled with acts of compassion and care, yet their hearts weighed down by an inexplicable emptiness. These are women who have dedicated themselves to nurturing their families, supporting their friends, even excelling in their careers, yet find themselves yearning for genuine connection and companionship.

Guess what? It's time to start serving yourself. Be good to yourself. You are your best-friend. Until you admit that and embrace it, you'll continue to struggle. I did it a long time ago. In my 50s, I told myself that I wasn't going to spend the rest of my adult life wishing and hoping for something or someone else. I decided to become that person. The status quo wasn't good enough for me.

We need to feel courageous enough to disrupt the status quo. By not disrupting it, we are automatically supporting it. If you have unfulfilled dreams but feel constricted about sharing them or even moving toward them, you may think you want to change the world, but your actions are showing something different. Disruption is how we change the world. Doing what others can't or won't do. Disruption is not as difficult or offensive and you might think. It's pretty much basically following your truth, unapologetically.

As women, there are a lot of things we've choked on over the years while being told to "get over it." Well, I'm over it. Too many women simply give up as they get older. It's just too hard to continue to push against conventional wisdom or "the way things are." I agree, it can feel difficult sometimes to break through all the bullshit. If you need convincing, or need help getting there, will you let me know?

Your needs come first. And, oh, the feeling of absolute freedom of being on the other side!

CHAPTER 11

You're Not a Bitch

Women back down too easily. We tend to be overly sensitive about what other people think.

Does your communication style sometimes land you in hot water? Do you fear that people might use the "B" word when describing you behind your back? Or maybe even to your face?!

I have a natural inclination towards directness in my communication style—I don't mince words; I tell it like it is. While this honesty serves me well in many situations, there are instances where it has led to some challenges. Yes, there have been occasions where my straightforwardness has rubbed people the wrong way or been perceived as too blunt. It's not that I intend to cause offense or discomfort, but rather that I value transparency, because that is what leaders do.

Does this make me a "bitch"?

Well, have you noticed that men who display assertive or dominant behavior are often praised and admired, rather than criticized or insulted? That feels like a double-standard to me. It highlights the unequal power dynamics and gender biases that persist in our society. While progress has been made in challenging and dismantling these stereotypes, the use of gendered insults continues to perpetuate harmful attitudes towards women. I try my best to recognize and challenge these biases in order to create a culture where a woman's voice can be heard.

Making your voice heard does not make you a "bitch".

We're not being THAT, so stop allowing people to say you ARE. You're not. You are being frank, sometimes with strong words and emotions. That's not the same thing. Don't you hate it when people beat about the bush and never get to the point? Well then, stop beating around the bush. Be straightforward. It's not mean-spirited, nor is it unreasonable. And just because someone judges you harshly for it does not mean that you deserved it. This might be their opinion of you, but opinion is not fact. Opinion and fact are not the same thing.

I find that women, when aggressively confronted, back down too easily. We tend to be overly sensitive about what other people think. We find ourselves entangled in the web of caring too much about others' perceptions of us. We walk a tightrope between valuing our own opinions and being overly sensitive to external judgments. This tendency to prioritize others' opinions over our own can lead us down a path where we begin to internalize external criticisms, mistaking them for objective truths. In doing so, we unintentionally undermine our self-confidence and diminish our sense of self-worth.

But a strong confident woman doesn't have to hide who she is. She doesn't allow people to continue to call her names or put her down or dismiss her ideas. She has a brain and can think for herself. She can state her own opinion.

However, as a woman who tries to advance herself and strives to be a leader, I've also seen first-hand how a well-intentioned but overly blunt remark can inadvertently hurt or alienate others, causing rifts in communication and straining connections. Therefore, I've made a conscious effort to guard my communication style, incorporating elements of empathy and consideration into my sometimes-too-straightforward approach. By carefully choosing my words and taking into account the feelings of those I'm communicating with, I've found that I can maintain my integrity while also nurturing positive and harmonious relationships. This ongoing process of balancing honesty with tact is not always easy, but I've come to recognize its immense value in fostering respect and mutual support.

However, I don't have to be reactive. That just shows weakness. I've come to recognize that finding the right balance between honesty and tact is essential in fostering positive relationships and effective communication. Sometimes there's a delicate dance between honesty and tact. While honesty is undeniably important for building trust and authenticity in relationships, I've learned that it must be accompanied by tact and sensitivity as well.

When going into a tense situation where conflict might arise, I try to be confident, strong, and assertive. But I also lean on my intuition and look for signs that my communication might be displaced.

Here are five ways a woman can go in strong, but also effectively:

- When expressing opinions or concerns, frame them using "I" statements to convey your perspective without assigning blame or making accusations. For example, instead of saying "You always do this wrong," try saying "I feel frustrated when things aren't done according to the plan."
- Demonstrate empathy and understanding by actively listening to the other person's viewpoint without interrupting or jumping to conclusions. Reflect back what they've said to ensure mutual understanding before expressing your own thoughts.
- When providing feedback or criticism, focus on specific behaviors or actions rather than making generalizations about the person's character. Be respectful and offer suggestions for improvement in a supportive and encouraging manner.
- Clearly communicate your boundaries and expectations in a firm but respectful manner. Use assertive language to express your needs without apologizing or feeling guilty for asserting yourself.
- Approach conflicts or disagreements with a willingness to find common ground and reach a mutually beneficial solution. Be open to listening to the other person's perspective and be prepared to negotiate and compromise to resolve differences peacefully.

Finally, and most importantly, don't allow anyone to take advantage of your emotions by calling you out for being the leader you are called to be. Here are the facts: You're a star! You're amazing! You're not a "bitch"! If you need to apologize for something you said or did, say "I'm sorry" and bounce back. Don't let THAT stop you from being the woman you were meant to be.

CHAPTER 12

Remember Who You Once Were

Just because you grew up doesn't mean that you can't reconnect with that little girl who once had boundless dreams.

Imagine walking down a bustling street, the air thick with the hustle and bustle of city life, when suddenly a familiar aroma drifts past your nostrils. In an instant, you are transported back to your childhood, a time when the world seemed vast and full of wonder.

Perhaps it's the scent of freshly baked cookies, wafting from a nearby bakery, that conjures images of your grandmother's kitchen—a haven of warmth and love where sweet treats awaited. Or maybe it's the earthy aroma of summer rain, reminiscent of carefree days spent splashing in puddles and chasing rainbows.

Catching a scent that evokes memories of childhood is like stumbling upon a hidden treasure buried deep in your mind. It's an unexpected journey back in time, a nostalgic embrace that reminds you that life was once simpler and that you still had dreams.

I love moments like this; they always surprise me. But they are also a jolt and maybe even conjure up some disappointment inside of me. What happened? Where did my dreams go?

Here's what I want you to do today.

Get away for a while, at least for an hour or so. Take a walk or do something else relaxing and sublime. Then pause for a moment and allow the gentle breeze of nostalgia to sweep you back to the tender years of your youth. Close your eyes and relish in the memories of boundless joy that once adorned your childhood.

Then grab a pen and write down questions about those memories and then the answers:

- What did you enjoy as a little girl?
- What were you especially good at?
- What were the simple pleasures that brought a smile to your lips?
- When did you feel especially proud?
- Who was your best friend and why?
- If adventure beckoned, what daring exploits would you undertake?
- What's your favorite childhood memory and why?
- Did you have dreams of who you wanted to be when you grew-up?

It might have been a long time since you've allowed yourself to remember some of these things. That's why I want you to think about them and write them down. One effective method I have discovered over the years is that if I get stuck and my creativity is stunted, it helps if I write a question and then answer it. You may think of other questions as well!

Let the ink flow freely as you immortalize these precious recollections, for within them lies the sacred key to finding "you" again. Recall with fondness the characteristics that defined your youthful spirit—the tenacity that fueled your pursuits, the compassion that warmed your interactions, and the resilience that carried you through life's trials.

Of course, not everything about our childhood was roses. Some of us even experienced deep trauma. But try to remember the time when you felt most innocent and dreamed big dreams. Try to remember the times when you didn't fear the present or the future, when you fully believed you could be anyone you wanted to be. For some of us, this might be an easy exercise, but for others it might be a little harder. That's OK. The important thing is to recollect that you once had unfulfilled dreams that you KNEW you could accomplish. You had no doubt about it.

Those are the memories I beg you to hold onto, to cradle in your heart, and to breathe back to life. Deep breaths. Breathe it in! For within them lies the essence of your truest self—the fearless, hopeful dreamer you were always meant to be.

Just because you grew up and life dealt you its fair share of setbacks and hardships, doesn't mean that you can't reconnect with that little girl who once gazed at the world with wide-eyed wonder and boundless dreams. You are still her! You can still be the younger version of yourself—full of innocence and unbridled enthusiasm. And though the years may have weathered your exterior and tempered your spirit, the core of who you are remains unchanged.

You are still that resilient, courageous little girl, capable of changing the world.

I want you to embrace your former self with open arms, welcome her back into your heart, and allow her boundless optimism to reignite the flames of possibility within you. Anything is still possible. The only thing that you cannot accomplish is what you believe is impossible. Take the blinders off and write out the answers to these questions. Think big. Think bold. Think up things that you might even be a bit embarrassed to tell anyone. You were born with unlimited potential and you still have unlimited potential.

When you begin to do this— and it won't be easy at first—you'll start to shed the heavy cloak of doubt and inhibition that weighs you down, and you'll feel the burdens of past disappointments and societal expectations fall away like autumn leaves. In their place will bloom a newfound sense of liberation, as you embrace the potential that has ALWAYS resided within the depths of your heart. It's time to throw away the self-doubt and be like the stars that shine so brightly.

The stars are eternally bright, and so are you!

CHAPTER 13

Stay Curious

Ladies, it's time to get curious again! It's time to redefine what it means to age with enthusiasm.

Amidst the hustle and bustle of a holiday family gathering, the atmosphere within our home was electric with the laughter and chatter of numerous children and grandchildren. With eight kids and step-kids, alongside an impressive count of twenty grandchildren, my abode was bursting at the seams with love and liveliness. I love the Christmas holidays!

However, amidst the joyful chaos, a small crisis emerged in the heart of our home—the kitchen. As pots clanged and the aroma of a sumptuous feast filled the air, a sudden gush of water disrupted the festivities. The kitchen sink, worn down by years of service, had decided to spring a leak, threatening to dampen not just the floor but also the spirits of our merry gathering. Bah! Humbug!

In a moment of both frustration and ingenuity, one of my sons took matters into his own hands. Amidst the clamor of the gathering, he made a bold decision: Rather than allowing the leak to persist and worsen, he swiftly ripped the faucet out entirely. A stop-gap effort that would only last for so long, I was left alone to fix it the next morning, something I'd never done before. But rather than find (and pay for) a plumber, I got curious.

So, I embarked on a journey to Home Depot, the bastion of DIY enthusiasts and home improvement aficionados. Upon arrival, I engaged in a conversation with one of the knowledgeable employees, seeking his advice on selecting the perfect replacement faucet for our kitchen. We navigated through the aisles, perusing an array of gleaming faucets, each promising to restore functionality and aesthetics to my beleaguered sink.

Armed with my newly acquired faucet and a determination to conquer the challenge at hand, I delved into the realm of online tutorials, scouring YouTube for a fix-it video that would guide me through the installation process. Then I went to work. With each twist of the wrench and each satisfying click of the new fixture into place, I felt a sense of accomplishment swell within me. I got the best of my curiosity. I told myself, "Now I've got another skill under my belt. I'm amazing!"

What's the point of my leaky faucet story?

I believe the older we get, the less curious we get. As we age, it's common to see the flame of curiosity dim and our appetite for adventure wane. The routine of daily life, coupled with years of responsibilities and obligations, can gradually erode our sense of wonder. For so many years it was go…go…go! We didn't have time to stop and smell the roses, right?

Moreover, the challenges we once faced head-on with gusto may start to appear daunting, leading us to shy away from problem-solving and innovation. While this phenomenon affects both men and women, it often seems to have a more pronounced impact on us women. Our culture can subtly influence women to prioritize stability over exploration and conformity over curiosity. As a result, women find themselves navigating a landscape where the pursuit of adventure and the thrill of solving problems take a back seat to more traditional roles and expectations.

Yet, I believe recognizing this trend is the first step towards reclaiming our innate sense of curiosity and adventure. Ladies, it's time to get curious again! It's time to challenge the status quo and redefine what it means to age with vigor and enthusiasm. Through intentional practices such as seeking out new experiences, embracing failure as a stepping stone to growth, and fostering a supportive community of like-minded individuals, women can reignite their curiosity and rediscover the joy of exploration. With determination and perseverance, we can break free from the constraints of societal norms and embark on a journey of self-discovery, empowerment, and limitless potential.

By now you know I like to ask you to write things down. So, grab a pen and answer these questions:

- How have societal expectations influenced my choices and behaviors regarding curiosity and adventure?
- Have I allowed fear of judgment or failure to hold me back from pursuing new experiences and challenges?
- In what ways has my upbringing and cultural background shaped my attitudes towards risk-taking and exploration?
- Do I prioritize stability and security over the excitement of stepping into the unknown?

- Have I internalized gender norms that discourage women from being adventurous or inquisitive?
- Have I become complacent in my comfort zone, avoiding opportunities for growth and learning?
- How do I view failure, and do I allow setbacks to deter me from trying new things?

My hope and prayer is that by asking yourself these questions, you'll begin to find ways to regain that sense of wonder, curiosity, and get-it-done attitude you once had. I know you once had it. We all did! It's a quality ingrained in every person, in every woman, and it can't go away regardless of the obstacles we've faced or the societal pressures we've endured.

I have absolute faith that within each woman that spirit still burns brightly, waiting to be reignited and reclaimed.

You are amazing!

CHAPTER 14

Your Random Thoughts Are Not Always So

Here's the problem: When we blame erratic emotions on menopause, it can get us into trouble.

Women, particularly women in menopause, experience a wide range of thoughts and emotions that can feel overwhelming or unpredictable. Random impulses seem to come out of nowhere and lead us to make decisions we later regret. They might occur in the form of something we say or how we react to someone.

Does that sound familiar?

It reminds me of when I once walked through a house of mirrors at a carnival. Walking through a house of mirrors can be a surreal experience. As I stepped inside, I was engulfed in a world of reflections stretching in every direction. It felt like being transported into another dimension where reality and illusion intertwined. With mirrors lining the walls on all sides, each turn I took revealed a new reflection of myself, fragmented and distorted in unexpected ways. Some reflections made me appear tall and elongated, while others made me seem short and squat. It was as if I was witnessing different versions of myself, each with its own quirks and characteristics.

Depending on your mindset, walking through a house of mirrors can evoke a range of emotions. Some may find it exhilarating, enjoying the novelty of seeing themselves reflected from different angles. Others may feel uneasy or anxious, struggling with the distorted reflections and the sense of being watched from all directions. I didn't really like it much, but it reminded me of myself and my random thoughts and emotions.

What if I told you that your thoughts and emotions are not as random as you might think? What if there was a way to better control them? Would you be interested?

Before I explain, let's acknowledge that menopause can leave women feeling profoundly unbalanced and disconnected from themselves due to hormonal fluctuations. It's simply biology, and sometimes we can't fight mother nature. The hormonal changes associated with menopause can disrupt mood regulation and cognitive function, leading to mood swings and cognitive symptoms like brain fog. Physical symptoms such as hot flashes and changes in libido can further exacerbate feelings of discomfort and disconnection from one's body. For some women, the hormonal imbalance is worse than others. And yes, that's random.

But we also need to recognize that our feelings, thoughts, dreams, or impulses are not as random as we might think. Instead, they are our most accurate information system. If we have shut them down, for whatever reason (and there are many), we are functioning like an airplane with one of our engines disabled.

Random thoughts often seem to arise spontaneously, but they are rarely as random as they appear. Instead, they are deeply rooted in our background, experiences, upbringing, and surroundings. Our thoughts are influenced by a myriad of factors, including cultural influences, personal beliefs, past traumas, and learned behaviors. For example, a seemingly random thought may be triggered by a familiar scent, a fleeting memory, or a subconscious association with a past experience. These underlying factors shape our perceptions, biases, and thought patterns, guiding the trajectory of our thoughts in ways that may not always be immediately apparent.

Here's the problem for women: When we blame erratic emotions on menopause, it can get us into trouble. When we blame them on the past or our current surroundings or predicament, it can also get us into trouble. We say and do things we probably shouldn't.

What's the solution?

By recognizing the interconnectedness of our thoughts with our lived experiences, we can gain insight into ourselves and better understand the motivations behind our actions and reactions.

Blaming emotions solely on menopause or external circumstances can oversimplify the complexity of human emotions and potentially lead to misunderstandings or misinterpretations. While menopause and external factors, like past experiences or current surroundings, can certainly influence emotions, they are just one piece of the puzzle. Emotions are multifaceted and can be influenced by a combination of biological, psychological, and social factors.

It's essential to take a holistic approach to understanding and managing emotions, acknowledging the interplay between internal and external factors. This involves self-reflection, emotional awareness, and cultivating healthy coping mechanisms to navigate with resilience and grace through the ups and downs of life. By recognizing the nuanced nature of emotions, women can empower themselves to take ownership of their emotional well-being and foster healthier relationships with themselves and others.

Take some time to rediscover yourself. Introduce yourself to yourself! Get curious with you. The next time you experience an unwanted, intrusive emotion or reaction, sit down and ask yourself these seven questions. It always helps to write down your answers.

- Where did I first encounter this belief or feeling?
- Have I examined this belief critically, or have I accepted it without question?
- Does this belief align with my values and principles?
- How does this belief or feeling impact my behavior and decisions?
- Have I considered alternative perspectives or interpretations?
- How might my cultural background or upbringing influence this belief?
- What would it mean for me if I were to change or let go of this belief?

Before you take the cork off and explode, remind yourself that you are in control of you. Random isn't always random. The difference between you and an actual star-turned-supernova, is that you have a choice to shine. For a star, that process is a natural explosion of unimaginable beauty. For you, as a human, you often have a choice.

You are the star of your life!

CHAPTER 15

Redefine Your Golden Years

The best time to change the world is later in life. We have more wisdom and we have less to lose.

Someone once told me they were looking forward to their "golden years." I winced. What if all women simply slowed down in their 50s and then retired in the 60s? What would that look like? I'm not against getting a little rest and relaxation, but putting life on permanent pause?

My friend, Dr. Jo Anne Lyon, is the founder of World Hope International and served as the first CEO, overseeing the mission to alleviate poverty, suffering, and injustice around the world.

During her tenure as World Hope's CEO, Jo Anne brought a strong focus on the role of faith, regarding women's inclusion, to her involvement with several countries experiencing fragility, conflict, and violence. I've traveled with Joanne, working with World Hope in some of the world's most dangerous places.

She's in her 80s now, but in her 50s, she started her powerful, world-changing organization. You read that correctly: In her 50s! Since then, she's received seven honorary doctorates, invitations from more than one U.S. President, and appointments to several boards where her expertise and knowledge are revered. She once told me that she never even thought about her age when she founded World Hope. "We are called to change the world. We are called to overcome evil with good. There's no age when that stops," she said.

Jo Anne's tale of her harrowing journey through the heart of West Africa sent shivers down my spine.

When in Sierra Leone, surrounded by the deafening echoes of gunfire and the cries of the oppressed, she found herself leading a small group of doctors into the abyss of terror. With the weight of thousands of dollars strapped to her body, a heavy burden both physically and emotionally, Jo Anne knew that their mission was perilous. The RUF, a merciless force entrenched in the blood-soaked soil of Sierra Leone, held dominion over the country, leaving a trail of unimaginable horrors in their wake.

As she and the doctors attempted to navigate through the terrain, they were abruptly halted by the presence of armed soldiers. In that moment of dread, Jo Anne's gaze turned skyward, a silent plea escaping her lips as she sought divine intervention. With a prayer clinging to her lips, she steeled herself for what lay ahead, knowing that their fate rested in the hands of a higher power. They led her into a dungeon where she faced the very embodiment of terror.

But in the claustrophobic confines of the rebel stronghold, with nerves of steel, Jo Anne dared to negotiate with the warlords. Every word uttered was a delicate thread, a lifeline hanging above the abyss of destruction. Yet, against all odds, a miracle unfolded amidst the chaos. Through the sheer force of her will and unwavering determination, Jo Anne secured the impossible—a safe passage through the heart of enemy territory where she could help the victims of the war.

When will Jo Anne retire? She shakes her head when people mention that she should retire. She explains that around the world, there is no retirement age in non-western countries. "We've been socialized in the U.S.A. to think that way because we have adequate resources to be able to do that. Our culture has told us that we need to stop at a certain age." She says her calling, to alleviate poverty, suffering, and injustice around the world, never had a time limit or a retirement plan.

In a world where the echoes of inequality still reverberate, the presence of women is not merely a necessity but a LIFELINE. I think the notion of retirement for women is a luxury that society cannot afford; for their wisdom, experience, and resilience are invaluable assets in the ongoing battle for gender equality. Instead of stepping back, women must continue to stride forward, their footsteps paving the way for future generations. To retire is to relinquish our position of influence, a position from which one can uplift and empower other women. The cost of retirement transcends personal comfort; it is a relinquishment of responsibility, a tacit acceptance of the continued victimization of women.

Am I saying you should descend into dungeons with warlords? Am I saying you should risk your life to help women traumatized by war? No, not necessarily. But I am saying that we as women can change the world. And the best time to change the world is later in life. We have more wisdom and we have less to lose. Maybe our "golden years" should not be a time to look back, but look forward, a time to be Supernova women.

Are you ready to help change the world? Join me!

CHAPTER 16

Who Said You Should Retire?

No specific age is a finish line; it's a starting point for a fulfilling and dynamic second act.

When my husband retired and we moved from Japan back to the United States, I wasn't quite ready to sit on the rocking chair on the front porch. I had just turned 56 years old. Even though I had considered retiring as well, internally I was still active, my mind was still quick, and my body was cooperating. So why quit?

You might be ready to kick back and enjoy more leisure time, but you don't have to be. This might be the time for an exciting new chapter in your life. Don't let anyone tell you that you're too old. I certainly didn't.

For women, especially, this milestone can mark a new chapter of possibilities rather than an endpoint. With advancements in healthcare, shifting societal norms, and a growing recognition of the value of diverse perspectives in the workplace, women are empowered to continue thriving in their careers well beyond traditional retirement age. At 56, many women find themselves at the peak of their professional abilities, armed with decades of experience, wisdom, and skills honed through years of dedication.

Did you know that renowned chef, author, and television personality Julia Child rose to fame with her groundbreaking cookbook *Mastering the Art of French Cooking* and became a beloved TV figure in her late 50s? Grandma Moses started painting in her 70s. Nancy Pelosi was 66 years old when she ran for

Speaker of the House. Margaret Thatcher was Prime Minister of England at age 64.

Is this you too? If so, rather than slowing down, get ready to embrace new challenges, pursue passions, and make meaningful contributions as an employee, or maybe better yet, as a business owner. No specific age is a finish line; it's a starting point for a fulfilling and dynamic second act in one's career.

There's more than one reason not to retire:

1. First, continuing to work provides financial security, allowing you to maintain your independence and support yourself financially. In an era where retirement savings may not be enough to sustain a comfortable lifestyle, staying in the workforce can bolster savings and ensure a more stable financial future.
2. Second, work offers a sense of purpose and fulfillment, providing opportunities for personal growth, social interaction, and intellectual stimulation. Many older women derive satisfaction from contributing their skills and knowledge to their profession or community.
3. Finally, staying engaged in the workforce can help combat feelings of isolation and loneliness that some individuals may experience in retirement.

Since I had a license as a Marriage and Family Therapist from earlier in my career, I made the decision to re-launch. Every practice I set up over the years was a new adventure, with new challenges, new clientele, and new specialties. It was always fun and stimulating. So, I decided to set up a new practice not far from where we moved to the foothills of the Blue Ridge Mountains in Virginia, in a picturesque town called Warrenton.

It seemed like an easy decision— at first. But there were lots of challenges and I second-guessed my decision more than once. Did I know enough local people? Would I find my niche? Was the town big enough to support my practice? And the biggest question: Was I too old to start a new business? Also, owning a business as a woman can present unique challenges. Women entrepreneurs, compared to their male counterparts, often face disparities in access to funding and resources such as encountering hurdles in securing startup capital, loans, and venture capital investment. Additionally, gender bias can manifest in various forms, from stereotypes about leadership capabilities to discrimination in business dealings and negotiations.

Do you think I gave in? You guessed it. Not a chance! As a woman in her late 50s, I made it work. I convinced the local newspaper to write a story about my new practice, I got involved in the local Chamber of Commerce, and I bought some advertisements in a local magazine. Before long, one-by-one, women came knocking at my door.

Marianne, my marriage is in trouble! Can you help?

Marianne, I'm struggling with my career choices. Can you offer some guidance?

Marianne, I'm feeling overwhelmed with my financial situation. Can you provide some advice?

Marianne, I'm having difficulties managing stress and anxiety. Can you suggest coping strategies?

Marianne, I'm worried about my aging parents' health. Can you offer support or resources?

Marianne, I'm grappling with a difficult decision and could use an outside perspective. Can you lend an ear?

I must have given my clients good advice because they kept coming back, and they spread the word. My fledgling practice grew and grew, and I had to add interns, staff, and more office space. I could hardly keep up. And imagine me at age 66. Believe it or not, the Chamber of Commerce eventually asked me to become Chairman!

Enough about me though. My point is this: If you're approaching retirement age or you're at or past retirement age, you don't have to quit. You can begin again or for the very first time. You might be entering the most productive time of your life, so don't let everyone around you pressure you to slow down. You may find yourself on the cusp of your most remarkable chapter yet, where experience meets innovation and wisdom fuels audacity!

CHAPTER 17

Envision Your Funeral to Live Again

Reflecting on the inevitable cycle of life isn't an act of morbidity but an acknowledgment of our mortality.

My friend Susan and I met when we were expats in Tokyo, where we became fast friends. We had lots of fun together, both as couples with our husbands and also as girlfriends. We even climbed Mt. Fuji together. So, when I heard she was diagnosed with terminal, stage-4 colorectal cancer, I was really hurting for her and I went to visit.

She and I sat together in silence for a while. She looked me in the eye, telling me how much she valued our friendship and the wonderful life we had shared as friends. Then she said, "I have to tell you something. I'm not afraid." That's when the tears started to run down my cheeks. Susan was a woman who radiated a wonderful feeling of *joie de vivre*. Always game, always fun, always interested. "I've had such a wonderful life, and I feel almost perfect. I have nothing to complain about, and I'm not afraid." The fact that she knew I needed to hear that and she needed to say it, shows the kind of brave and insightful person she is.

Susan will leave a lasting legacy for sure. She has always had a "yes" mentality towards life. She has embraced opportunities for travel and adventure. She has loved her family and her friends and has a regular practice and lifestyle of gratitude, generosity, and strong faith. All these things and who Susan has been over the years have built a foundation that gives her the added support, resilience, hope, and courage to live each day as it comes with no fear of the future and no regrets.

The older you get, the more you'll experience around you sickness, pain, and yes, death. You'll attend more funerals as well. This is a fact of life. It's always sad, and it serves as a poignant reminder of the preciousness of life. It also instills a sense of urgency inside of me. When I leave a funeral, part of me screams, "Not yet…I need more time!"

Sometimes I envision my own funeral. Does that sound morbid to you? It shouldn't. The circle of life includes our eventual passing. Reflecting on the inevitable cycle of life isn't an act of morbidity but rather an acknowledgment of our mortality. Just as the seasons change and the flowers bloom only to fade, so too do our lives follow a natural course. I think embracing this reality allows us to live more fully in the present, cherishing each moment and nurturing the relationships that mean so much to us. It's a reminder to make the most of our time on this earth, to leave behind a legacy. So, while envisioning my own funeral may seem unconventional, it serves as a gentle reminder to embrace the beauty and impermanence of life, embracing every precious moment!

Do you ever wonder what your friends and loved ones will say about you at your funeral?

They might speak about the passions and pursuits that defined you: What were your greatest accomplishments and contributions? What were your core values and beliefs? How did you inspire and influence those around you? They might also ponder the nature of your relationships and connections: Who were the most important people in your life? How did you nurture and support your loved ones? What memories and experiences did you share with them? They might also consider the broader impact you had on your community and the world: What causes were you passionate about? How did you give back and make a difference? What will be your lasting imprint on the lives of others? Ultimately, these questions serve as a reflection of the multifaceted aspects of your identity and the profound influence you had during your time on earth.

Some of these questions might be answered in your obituary or during your eulogy. Do you like to read obituaries? I do. For the same reasons I sometimes think about my own funeral, I think there's a certain fascination in glimpsing the snapshots of lives lived—the stories of triumph, love, and resilience, all captured in a few concise paragraphs. Each obituary is a tribute to a unique individual, a testament to their journey through this world. To me, it's a celebration of the human experience in all its complexity. In those brief passages, we find echoes of our own hopes, fears, and dreams. We connect with the shared threads of humanity that bind us all together, reminding us of the fleeting nature of life and the importance of cherishing every moment.

I also wonder who will write my obituary. Who will say my eulogy? But it's dawned on me that I am the author of my obituary and the giver of my eulogy. It's my life and I'm the only one who can truly control what people will think about me and what they will say when I'm gone.

It's important that you see life this way. You control your destiny, your legacy. Every action, every choice that you make contributes to the narrative of who you are and how you will be remembered. Yes, there will be moments of imperfection, times when you stumble or fall short of your ideals. But it's in those moments of vulnerability that the richness of your story lies. After all, it's not the absence of mistakes that defines us but rather how we rise from them, how we grow, learn, and evolve as women.

I want you to take a few minutes sometime soon to write down your obituary, or if you're up to it, write your own eulogy. Stephen Covey, the author of *7 Habits of Highly Effective People*, calls it an "aspirational eulogy." Covey once famously encouraged individuals to envision the eulogy they would want delivered at their own funeral—one that went beyond mere accomplishments and accolades, delving into the core of their character, values, and impact on others. This exercise served as a powerful reminder of the importance of living in alignment with one's deepest principles and aspirations.

When you write it down, it will help you to decide the significance of prioritizing what truly matters the most to you, fostering meaningful relationships, and leaving behind the legacy you want remembered. It will serve as a gentle nudge to seize the opportunities before you, to mend broken ties, to express love and gratitude, and to make a meaningful impact in the world while you still have the chance. It will keep you focused on how you want to be remembered.

Me?

There are many things I want to be remembered for: a wife, a mom, a grandmother, a friend. But I also want to be remembered as a woman who helped other women find their calling, as someone whose heart was dedicated to extending a compassionate hand to women who face adversity and trauma across the globe by offering solace, understanding, and resources to help them heal and reclaim their strength. Whether through mentorship, coaching, counseling, activism, or philanthropy, I want to be remembered as the woman whose impact had a ripple effect of empowerment and compassion that continues to resonate through the lives of women everywhere. A Supernova woman!

You? Write it down!

CHAPTER 18

Be Your Own Hero

As women, we've been conditioned to believe that our happiness hinges on finding someone or something else.

I'm not going to lie. There are times when I wish someone would show up at my door with chocolate, a bouquet of flowers, a hot cup of coffee...and one million dollars. Oh, and a hug. Wouldn't it be nice if a knight in shining armor would swoop in and fix everything? Or a charming prince who knew our every thought and took care of our every need?

I think it's every woman's fantasy, and it goes all the way back to our childhood.

Remember the whimsical realm of Disney-inspired narratives of the girl who waited for her prince to come? Picture a charming village nestled in a picturesque valley, where cobblestone streets wind past quaint cottages adorned with colorful blooms. Here she lives in a quaint little cottage at the edge of town. She spends her days dreaming of the fabled Prince Charming who will one day sweep her off her feet. She gazes wistfully out of her window, her imagination ablaze with visions of grand ballrooms and gallant knights. She tends to her chores with a song in her heart, her mind wandering to thoughts of her elusive prince. She waits, and waits, and waits. But alas, days turn into weeks, and weeks into months, and months into years, yet Prince Charming remains but a figment of her imagination.

Sounds familiar, right?

If you're still waiting for your hero to show up or your situation to change, I have a message for you:

He's not. She's not. Whatever and whoever you're waiting for, isn't coming.

It's a hard truth to swallow, isn't it? For years women have been fed the narrative that someday, somehow, Prince Charming will ride in on his noble steed and sweep us off our feet, solving all our problems with a single kiss. But here's the reality check: life just doesn't work that way.

As women, we've been conditioned to believe that our happiness and fulfillment hinge on finding someone or something else. We've been taught to wait because we're not good enough on our own. But the truth is, the only person capable of saving you is staring back at you in the mirror. Mirror, mirror on the wall, you ARE the fairest one of all!

One of the empowering things you can do as a woman is to shatter your own fairy tale illusions and embrace a new reality: You are the heroine of your own story. You hold the power to shape your destiny, to conquer your fears, and to build the life you've always dreamed of. No knight in shining armor required. When you stop looking for love in all the wrong places and begin to understand that there is no savior coming, no white knight, you discover that she is already here.

She's YOU!

You have everything you need inside of you to make your life better, happier, more fulfilling; your relationships more authentic; and your bank account increased. You simply need to learn how to be your own hero.

I know it's hard. Life doesn't always turn out the way it should. Of course you're angry, and you have every right to be angry, hurt, betrayed, scared. Acknowledge your feelings and validate that they are normal. But don't stay there. Don't wallow in them. Don't let them ruin your day, week, or life. If you are not currently in the habit of talking kindly to yourself, start this moment. Learn to validate yourself. Tell yourself you love you.

Yes, of all the people that you need to love you, you are the most important and necessary. If you don't love yourself, you can't really, unconditionally, love anyone else. In some capacity you will criticize them and be hard on them like you are hard on yourself. Even unintentionally, simply because it's become a habit. Be kind to everyone, but first and foremost, be kind to YOU. This might be a new normal for you, especially if you feel like you've been the one doing the giving for so many years. But now it's time to get on the receiving end.

How does that work?

Here's a secret: Start to give yourself little treats. Don't deny treating yourself because you think you don't deserve it for one reason or another, or maybe you just don't take the time. Want some chocolate? Go get some. A bubble bath? Go turn the hot water on. Read a book, take a long walk, look up at the stars. Nurture yourself. Love yourself.

I like to keep a list of things that make me happy, so when I get in a funk and can't think of anything, I can pick something from my list. Simple things: pet my dogs, go outside and take a breath of fresh air, buy myself flowers, take myself out to lunch, have a cup of tea, see my kids and grandkids. If they are not close by, I can look at their photos. I can even take a break and watch a funny show, or take a nap, or listen to meditation music. Treat yourself like you really DO love you!

And what about your unfulfilled dreams?

You have dreams and goals that you think will make your life better. All women do, and that's awesome. Remember, you are a co-creator. You create the life you want. No one else can or will do it for you. Don't let your dreams and goals just hang in the air like some pipe dream that will never happen. Of course, it won't happen if you just dream about it and talk about it but never really expect it to materialize.

Your thoughts and feelings are powerful and even more powerful when they have a plan behind them. I'm here to tell you that there is nothing beyond your reach if you are willing to focus your thoughts, your energy, your emotions, and your actions. Believe in yourself, even if you think no one else does. Believe in your dreams and their ability to come true. You are created to create, to expand, and to grow. You have the spirit of your Creator inside of you and everything that He is, you are.

Unfortunately, over the years, we are conditioned to fit in, follow the rules, and not make waves. That of course is just so that everyone around you can be comfortable. But the truth is, you were not created to fit in, to keep quiet, and to not make waves. You were created to shine, to inspire others with your ideas and your growth and adventures and successes.

It's time to write your own princess story, one where the princess stops waiting around and starts creating the life of her dreams!

CHAPTER 19

You're Stronger Than You Think

Stop believing you are alone. You are alone because you have chosen to be alone.

I climbed a mountain yesterday, a mountain in Shenandoah National Park. It was tough, but with each step I conquered the mountain, pushing myself higher, and soaking in the breathtaking views on the way, especially at the summit. What a great feeling at the top! The experience left me invigorated and it reminded me of the strength I possess to tackle my obstacles.

Women are stronger than they're given credit for, right?

The experience also reminded me of what women frequently tell me during a coaching or counseling session. They will often complain to me that they feel alone in their struggle. "Often" might not actually be the most appropriate word because almost *every* woman tells me this. In fact, I've never had a woman tell me they don't feel some sense of loneliness.

Yes, as women, we often find ourselves feeling alone when facing towering mountains, seemingly insurmountable obstacles that loom before us, casting shadows of doubt and uncertainty. These mountains take on many forms—career challenges, relationship struggles, health concerns, financial burdens—and they can appear unique to each of us. But what if I told you that these mountains we face are not as different as they seem? What if I told you that every woman, regardless of her background or circumstance, is climbing *the same mountain*?

One of the most common misconceptions we hold is that our problems are unique, that no one else could possibly understand the challenges we face. But the truth is that while the details of our struggles may differ, the emotions they evoke—fear, doubt, frustration—are universal. Whether we're grappling with a difficult career decision or navigating the complexities of a relationship, we all experience moments of uncertainty and vulnerability. All women wrestle with the same demons that whisper doubt in our ears and threaten to derail our progress.

Stop believing you are alone. You are alone because you have chosen to be alone. That's a tough pill to swallow, but it's true. No woman needs to climb mountains by herself, nor should she try.

Do this: Imagine yourself alone in front of a mountain, preparing to climb it by yourself. Then imagine yourself in front of the same mountain, but this time with a group of other women who are preparing to climb it with you. Those two images, one by yourself and another with a group of women, leaves you with two very different emotions, right? Alone or together?

When I climbed that mountain, I climbed with a group of friends. We each had our own individual climb, but we had each other. We had cheerleaders, coaches, mentors, and friends on the way up. Yes, we were each responsible for our own individual steps, but we supported each other to the top. We also celebrated together on the summit.

As we each embark on our midlife journey, it's essential to recognize that while our paths may diverge, the essence of the mountain climb remains the same. Just as no two snowflakes are alike, no two women's experiences are identical. Yet, beneath the surface, we are bound by a shared experience, the same mountain.

Why do we often try to climb by ourselves?

Women often find themselves inclined to tackle challenges alone due to societal pressures and ingrained beliefs about independence and self-sufficiency. From a young age, many of us are conditioned to believe that asking for help is a sign of weakness, leading us to internalize the idea that we must handle everything on our own. Additionally, historical and cultural norms have perpetuated the myth of the "superwoman," portraying women as capable of effortlessly juggling multiple roles without assistance. Consequently, seeking support from others can sometimes be viewed as an admission of failure or inadequacy, prompting women to carry the weight of their burdens silently.

Nothing can be further than the truth. So rather than climbing a mountain by yourself, why don't you look for and invite other women to climb with you? Why go solo? Maybe the problem is not your mountain, but the fact that you think you're by yourself.

Girlfriends, the answer lies not in trying to climb the mountain alone but in finding the strength and resilience to climb it together. No, we cannot control the obstacles that life throws our way, but we can control how we respond to them. We can choose to embrace the challenges before us, to view them not as barriers but as opportunities for growth and transformation. Together, we're better.

Think about it: In the world of mountain climbing, camaraderie and teamwork are absolutely essential elements for reaching the summit. Whether it's sharing equipment, offering encouragement during difficult stretches, or providing support in times of crisis, the bonds formed between climbers are often what make the difference between success and failure. Each member of the team plays a crucial role, contributing their unique skills and strengths to the collective effort. In the face of extreme conditions and unforeseen obstacles, climbers must trust in their companions and work together harmoniously to ascend to the top.

Life is the same way, so as we ascend higher and higher, inching closer to the summit with each step, we may stumble and falter along the way. We may face setbacks and obstacles that threaten to knock us off course. But it is in these moments of adversity that our true strength is revealed, as we draw upon the strength of other women in our lives.

And when, at last, we stand triumphantly atop the mountain, gazing out at the breathtaking vista before us, we will realize that the journey was never about reaching the summit alone. It was about the lessons we learned from each other along the way, the friendships we forged, and the transformation that took place within us. It was about discovering that, despite our perceived differences, we are all climbing the same mountain, facing the same challenges, and striving toward the same goal of self-empowerment and fulfillment.

Together, we will conquer the mountain, one step at a time, until we reach the summit and beyond!

CHAPTER 20

Don't Make the Little Things Too Big

Women are famous for magnifying flaws or mistakes, even when others may scarcely notice.

The trauma of war in Sierra Leone, West Africa, showed me that so many of my problems, or my perceived problems, weren't problems at all. My internal magnifying lens was broken. It was a lesson I'll never forget and a constant reminder to find something bigger than myself when I'm feeling overwhelmed.

Women, like anyone, can internalize and fixate on things that may seem small and insignificant to others but carry a heavy weight in their own minds. From societal standards of appearance to personal relationships and professional endeavors, women face a multitude of pressures that can amplify their focus on seemingly minor details.

These internalized pressures can lead to feelings of inadequacy or anxiety, driving a relentless pursuit of perfection in various aspects of life. Moreover, the fear of judgment or failure can exacerbate this tendency, causing women to dwell on perceived flaws or mistakes, regardless of their actual significance in the grand scheme of things.

I think it's fair to say we learned to do this as little girls. From a young age, we compared ourselves to others, a behavior influenced by a multitude of factors including societal norms, peer interactions, and media portrayals. We learned to stuff and internalize messages that suggested our value was tied to external factors such as appearance, talents, or achievements, leading to constant comparison with our peers. We made a big deal about little things.

Later in life, when we "grow up" we learn not to, most of the time. But we still occasionally find ourselves ensnared in the trap of internalizing trivial matters that should hold little significance. Yes, even grown women are famous for magnifying perceived flaws or mistakes, even when others may scarcely notice. While it's natural to strive for excellence, dwelling excessively on minutiae can detract from more meaningful pursuits and hinder personal growth.

I didn't even realize how much I was a victim of my own thoughts until I was invited on a trip to Sierra Leone, where I'd work with amputee victims and former child soldiers who were traumatized by war. It was the kind of experience that peels your heart open.

I was invited to help victims of brutal amputations deal with the trauma of their experiences. The stories I heard were heartbreaking and almost surreal. They were difficult to get my head around.

Listening to a mom describe how she was forced to sit and watch her six children shot before her very eyes, a man forced to watch his wife get brutally raped, story after story of how people were held down with their arms— or lips, legs, noses, or more— against a tree while the rebel soldiers hacked them off. Hearing the devastating tale of a child soldier as he spoke of how he was abducted and forced to join the rebel army at the threat of his own life. These stories still echo in my mind and heart.

Child soldiers in Sierra Leone represent a tragic chapter in the nation's history, where thousands of young boys and girls were forcibly recruited into armed groups during the brutal civil war that ravaged the country. Some, as young as seven, committed unspeakable atrocities: killing parents and siblings, assaulting neighbors, torching the villages they once called home. Some were forced to serve as sex slaves. Many were injected with drugs to curb their inhibitions against committing violence. Once the killing ended, peace treaties were signed and emergency humanitarian missions pulled out. But these children's trauma and sorrows persist.

Sitting down to talk with these people is a deeply sobering experience. Their stories are marked by unimaginable hardships and profound loss. The scars of war are etched into their memories, haunting their present-day realities. They suffer from nightmares, intense sadness, intrusive thoughts, and recurring violent images. Not surprisingly, these children who committed extreme acts of violence or were its victims, suffer the most persistent emotional health problems. Frequently, these children have difficulty with relationships after their release. They struggle with horrible guilt and shame. They are labeled as untrustworthy, which, in a vicious circle, deepens their sense of isolation. In their home communities, they are blamed for having destroyed the lives and property of the people they loved and lived with.

Girls face a compound burden. They are more likely to suffer more severe depression, anxiety, and PTSD compared with boys. Some returned to their communities having had unwanted pregnancies during their times with rebel groups. At home, they face the double stigma of having participated in violence and being seen as "impure," regardless of their war experiences.

Frankly, the trauma was so deep that it was hard to imagine I could help. But I believe that my words, my presence, and my prayers made a difference. At the very least, they were able to talk about it. And as we all know, talking about our trauma helps.

Perhaps the most profound lesson I learned on these trips was the concept of forgiveness. I listened as many of the victims spoke of how they forgave their attackers. The very idea that these innocent people could forgive the ones who victimized them was sobering to me.

Knowing how forgiveness releases the venom that can build up from hate and resentment, I realized how vital it is for true healing.

Leading a group of victims who were surprisingly able to confront one of their attackers, whose feelings and responses were obviously blunted by drugs, I watched as one by one they looked into his glassy, deadened eyes and said, "I forgive you." The forgiveness freed them. I never found out if the soldier was ever able to forgive himself.

When I returned from my trip, so many of the trivial things I was obsessed about disappeared. They all seemed so insignificant. It gave me perspective. Witnessing firsthand the resilience and resourcefulness of people living in such challenging circumstances provided a powerful reality check. It reminded me that I take so much for granted. It also served as a reminder of the resilience of the human spirit and the capacity to find joy and meaning amidst adversity. While my problems didn't disappear, the experience introduced me to something bigger than myself.

Take a few moments to reflect on the little things that become so big in your mind. These are things that can cause you to be depressed and anxious, and for no reason other than you let them. Then begin looking for opportunities to gain perspective. You might not sit down with war-torn victims like I did, but there are opportunities all around us to put our problems in their place. I promise it will lift your spirits, and of course, the spirits of those you help as well.

CHAPTER 21

Deconstruct Your Self-Limiting Narrative

Despite a desire for change, ingrained beliefs can prevent you from breaking free.

Skydiving for the first time is an intense mix of anticipation, fear, and exhilaration. Standing at the open door, the world below seems both impossibly distant and incredibly close. The leap into freefall is a rush of adrenaline, with senses overwhelmed by the wind's roar and the surreal sensation of weightlessness.

How do I know? I did it!

"But why, Marianne," you ask? I asked myself that same question when I jumped out of the airplane. But by the time I reached the ground, it all came together for me. Let me explain.

As a therapist and coach specializing in counseling women, particularly those over the age of 50, I observed a recurring pattern that I like to call "stuckness." It's a phenomenon where women find themselves entrenched in core beliefs that act as sticky traps, hindering their personal growth and fulfillment. These beliefs, often deeply ingrained over years of societal conditioning, familial influences, and personal experiences, create invisible barriers that hold them back from being happy.

For example, I've encountered women who cling to beliefs such as "I'm not good enough," or "I should always put others first," or "It's too late for me to change." These beliefs act as powerful anchors, keeping them tethered to past narratives and preventing them from embracing their true selves. Despite their desire for change and transformation, the pull of these ingrained beliefs can be incredibly strong, like a leash, making it challenging to break free.

Helping women recognize and address these core beliefs became a crucial aspect of my work. I supported them in unraveling layers of conditioning, and together we challenged their outdated beliefs, cultivating more self-awareness and more empowering narratives that align with their aspirations. By loosening the grip of these sticky beliefs, I saw women become

"unleashed." It was so much fun seeing them find happiness as they charted a new course for their lives.

What does this have to do with my jumping out of an airplane?

I came to the profound realization that I, too, had constructed my own set of self-limiting narratives, some of which had been woven into the fabric of my identity for many years. Despite the strides I had made in my personal and professional life, I found myself ensnared in patterns of thought that stifled my growth and potential. It was a humbling recognition that, despite my role as a guide and mentor to others, I was not immune to the influence of these self-imposed limitations.

Looking back, I saw how I had allowed the opinions and expectations of others to shape my sense of self-worth and possibility. Whether it was seeking validation from external sources or adhering to societal norms and expectations, I realized that I had often relinquished my autonomy, allowing others to define who I was and what I was capable of achieving.

In doing so, I unwittingly confined myself within a narrow framework of possibility, unable to fully embrace my potential.

Recognizing the parallels between my own struggles and those of the women I counsel was a profound moment of clarity. Just as I encourage my clients to challenge the narratives that hold them back, I understood the importance of confronting my own self-limiting beliefs head-on. So that's what I did. I confronted myself and as a symbolic act of taking off the leash, I decided to jump out of an airplane. I didn't let being a grandmother of 20 stop me!

Yes, it was terrifying. But I wanted to show myself, and other women, that they could let go.

Indeed, jumping out of an airplane was my way of symbolizing a woman's journey of letting go of the core beliefs that have held her back. When I stood at the door of that plane, I confronted all my fears and doubts, akin to confronting my deeply ingrained beliefs. My big leap into the sky represented my act of courageously stepping into the unknown, letting go of the familiar. And as I fell toward earth, I felt an incredible sense of liberation and weightlessness, mirroring my newfound freedom!

If you find yourself intrigued by the idea of taking that leap of faith, I wholeheartedly encourage you to consider experiencing the exhilaration of skydiving firsthand. It's an opportunity to confront your fears, challenge your limits, and embrace the sheer thrill of defying gravity. However, if the thought of jumping out of an airplane sends shivers down your spine (and believe me, it's not for everyone!), know that I did it not just for myself but also as a symbolic gesture for women everywhere who may feel trapped by their own self-limiting beliefs.

My decision to take that leap was driven by a desire to show solidarity with those who may be struggling to break free from the confines of their own minds. It's a testament to the resilience and courage of women everywhere who are on a journey of empowerment.

Whether you choose to soar through the skies or find your own path to liberation, know that you're not alone. I did it for you, for every woman who dares to dream beyond the constraints of convention and forges her own new path.

CHAPTER 22

Bored? Then Get Busy!

A slower pace offers opportunities for relaxation, but can also bring feelings of loneliness and isolation.

When my husband and I returned to the United States from our time in Japan, I was just a few years into my 50s. We moved to a home near the Blue Ridge Mountains. The culture shock was extreme, to say the least, and it was a lesson in transitions.

Japan is renowned for its bustling cities and vibrant culture. From the crowded streets of Tokyo to the lively markets of Osaka, the country is teeming with people going about their daily lives. The pace of life in Japan is often described as fast. Commuters pack into trains during rush hour, while neon lights illuminate the streets at night, showcasing the country's vibrant nightlife. Whether it's the hustle and bustle of shopping districts like Shibuya or the orderly chaos of Tsukiji Fish Market, Japan can be a sensory overload.

Our new home, back in America, was nestled in the woods near the Blue Ridge Mountains. It was very, very quiet. The rhythm of life slowed down amidst the solitude of the forest, providing a respite from the hustle and bustle of city living. Whether enjoying a stroll through the woods, picnicking by a brook, or simply unwinding on the porch while gazing at the star-studded night sky, one might find the setting idyllic. But frankly, for me it was a sudden jolt.

Now what should I do?

For many women after the age of 50, the transition from a busy, bustling life to one of relative calm and solitude can be profound. After decades of juggling multiple responsibilities, from careers to family obligations, they may find themselves suddenly confronted with an empty nest or retirement. The once constant noise and chaos of daily life are replaced by a newfound quietness that can feel eerily unfamiliar. While the slower pace offers opportunities for relaxation and self-reflection, it can also bring feelings of loneliness and isolation. That was me.

My friends told me to learn to adjust to this new chapter, to be patient and use it as a time of self-discovery. "Enjoy the quieter moments, Marianne," they all told me. I don't know about you, but I can only enjoy quiet moments for so long. I like to stay busy, and I like people, so it was unnatural for me to spend more time with birds than people.

I drove into "town" one morning, a town of no more than 20,000 people, but still in proximity to the Washington D.C. metro area. I walked up and down Main Street where the quaint setting was reminiscent of simpler times. But I wasn't quite ready for simpler times. I loved the town, but I was still young and not ready for retirement. As I walked up and down the sidewalks, I made a decision that would impact the lives of women all over my community. I decided to put my experience as a licensed marriage and family therapist to good use. I would rent some space off of Main Street and get to work!

Within a few months I opened a practice and began to find clients, mostly women who were just like me. They were in transition, dealing with a host of setbacks, issues, and yes, even trauma. They wanted change. They wanted to find renewed purpose and feel good about themselves. They didn't want to accept the roles society handed them. As women they wanted to feel valued. They wanted to make a difference! One by one, women would sit down in my office and share their feelings with me. We'd cry together and laugh together, and we found ways to chart a new course for their lives.

My practice grew rapidly as word spread. Women would search me out from the surrounding areas. I loved what I was doing. Not only was I keeping busy and finding a new sense of purpose for myself, but I was also helping other women do the same. The transition from Japan back to the United States was challenging, yes, but I didn't let it get the best of me. I learned to embrace the opportunity to adapt and evolve, recognizing that my passion for helping others and my commitment to personal growth were constants that transcended geographical boundaries. Rather than idly waiting by the brook, I dove headfirst into this new chapter of my life, eager to continue making a difference and embracing the opportunities that lay ahead.

My little practice eventually won awards. I was the fully engaged at our local Chamber of Commerce meetings. And all of this during a time when women were expected to sit back and watch. Not me. I took control of my life and helped a lot of other women do the same.

As a woman over 50, there may be moments when the desire to pause, rest, and reflect becomes enticing. After years of navigating the complexities of life, there's a natural inclination to crave stillness and tranquility. However, remember you don't have to stay there. Despite any perceived barriers, whether it be lack of experience, education, or the gap years spent away from the workforce, the drive to pursue one's passions should never be stifled. If the desire to get busy and dive into new ventures arises, then why not seize the opportunity? Every moment offers the chance to redefine oneself and chart a course toward fulfillment and success. So, if the heart whispers "go," then go forth boldly.

Want to get busy? Then get busy!

CHAPTER 23

Find Your Dory

You're not alone in feeling this way. But you have to reach out and ask for help.

Several years ago, I took a vacation certification course for scuba diving. Why not, right? I've watched scuba divers on TV, and it looks simple enough. Wrong!

Scuba diving is like stepping into an alien realm, encircled by darkness and the vast expanse of the ocean. Even though I was surrounded by other divers, I literally felt alone. The weight of unfamiliar gear and the sensation of breathing through a regulator felt suffocating, while the pressure and depth induced panic. My heart raced and the waves slapped me in the face.

As a therapist, I'm good at talking people down from anxiety and panic. But experiencing a panic attack while scuba diving is a terrifying ordeal that can quickly escalate in the underwater environment. As my heart raced and my breath became shallow, the feeling of suffocation intensified, exacerbated by the confined spaces and the weight of the gear. Panic set in as rational thought gave way to primal instincts of survival, leading to erratic movements and a desperate urge to get to the surface. The awareness of the depth and the potential dangers of rapid ascent only exacerbated my panic. This was no vacation!

One of the instructors, keenly attuned to the subtle signs of distress amidst the serene underwater landscape, noticed my struggle. She swiftly navigated through the water toward me, her presence reassuring me in the midst of my escalating panic. As she approached, her calm demeanor and steady gaze conveyed both empathy and authority, instilling hope amid my thoughts. With a gentle touch, she signaled for me to focus on her, guiding me to regulate my breathing in sync with hers. Her words, muffled by the water, carried a soothing tone, encouraging me to relax and trust in the training that had prepared me for this moment.

With her guidance, the intensity of the panic began to ebb, replaced by a sense of control and determination to overcome the challenge. In that fleeting encounter beneath the waves, her timely intervention became a testament to the invaluable role of experienced mentors in ensuring the safety and well-being of novice divers. We swam together for a few minutes while I calmed down and gathered my thoughts. I was still nervous, but in control, and able to begin to enjoy the beauty under the sea. We didn't swim for long but it gave me enough confidence to try again the next day.

When morning arrived, we were out at sea once again. This time I knew better what to expect, which is always a good thing. With the memory of the previous day's adventures still fresh in my mind, I felt a newfound sense of confidence. The uncertainties that had shrouded my initial dive had given way to some familiarity. Armed with that experience and more knowledge gained from the previous excursion, I approached the day's dive with a sense of anticipation rather than trepidation. My instructor offered me more help as well, calming my nerves and holding my hand as we dove into the depths. To this day, I remember how empowering it was for one woman to strengthen and encourage another to accomplish what we thought we could never do, hand-in-hand.

Remember Dory's famous line in the movie *Finding Nemo*, "just keep swimming!" That's exactly how I felt. With the gentle sway of seaweed and the kaleidoscope of marine life all around me, those words echoed in my mind like a mantra of determination. My scuba instructor was my Dory!

We all need a Dory. May I be your Dory?

Just as Dory's simple yet profound mantra "just keep swimming" echoed to me in the depths of the ocean, we all need encouragement and support. It fuels our determination to navigate the challenges of life with more courage and resilience. Much like Dory's endearing optimism and boundless enthusiasm, companionship and relationship with other women make us stronger.

Feeling alone as a woman, especially during midlife when children have grown and the home may feel quieter, is a sentiment we can all relate to. The transition into this phase of life can bring a mix of emotions, from pride in seeing children grow and flourish to a sense of emptiness or uncertainty about what comes next. In a society where roles and expectations often revolve around family and caregiving, finding oneself with more time and space can be disorienting. It's these moments of solitude that make you feel like you're scuba diving for the first time.

Amidst the confusion, don't panic. There's an opportunity for rediscovery, for reconnecting with passions, interests, and aspirations that may have been sidelined in the busyness of raising a family. But you can't do it alone. You need Dory. We all need Dory. Remember, you're not alone in feeling this way, and there's a world of possibilities waiting to be explored beyond the confines of your home. But you have to reach out and ask for help.

Guess what? There are scuba instructors all around us!

In the vast ocean of life, surrounded by the ebb and flow of experiences, there's a diverse community of women waiting to buoy you through the transitions of midlife. Among the waves, there are old friends, whose enduring presence serves as a comforting reminder of shared history and unwavering support. Therapists and counselors stand as beacons of guidance, offering a safe harbor for navigating the turbulent waters into self-discovery. Ministers and teachers provide wisdom and spiritual nourishment, illuminating the path forward with insights born of faith and knowledge.

Amidst it all, there's a multitude of women, each with her own story and strength, swimming alongside you. Some, with years of experience navigating the currents of life, extend a reassuring hand, ready to impart their wisdom and calm your nerves. With open hearts and outstretched hands, they invite you to join them, diving deep into the depths of your new life, exploring its depths and uncovering its hidden treasures. Together, this sisterhood of support forms a network of empowerment and encouragement, propelling you forward with confidence and grace as you navigate the ever-changing tides of midlife.

Need a hand but can't find one? You can always reach out to me too!

CHAPTER 24

Find Your Mountain to Climb

Stop listening to what other people say about what you can and can't do.

As a therapist and life coach, I am often told by women in midlife that it's too late to start over again, too late to experience anything new. Indeed, many women grapple with the idea that time is slipping away, leaving behind their unfulfilled dreams. What a depressing thought, right?

Societal narratives often dictate that by a certain age, opportunities for women dwindle, replaced by the monotony of routine. And yes, it's easy to succumb to the belief that the window for adventure is closing.

But this is nothing new if you're a woman. Society often imposes a myriad of limitations on women, dictating what they supposedly can't do based on gender norms and stereotypes. From early childhood, we're bombarded with messages about the roles we should fulfill and the paths we should follow. Whether it's being told we can't excel in certain professions, pursue ambitious goals, or express ourselves freely, the constraints imposed by societal expectations can feel suffocating!

I'm here to tell you: Stop listening to what other people say about what you can and can't do. Defy expectations, shatter glass ceilings, and rewrite the narrative of what is possible. The true essence of empowerment lies in challenging these imposed limitations, reclaiming autonomy over one's choices, and forging ahead despite the barriers society hands us. Women are not defined by what they can't do but by the resilience and determination with which they overcome obstacles.

Here's a profound truth: Life is not bound by age. Every moment presents a chance to embrace novelty, to chase passions, and to redefine what it means to flourish. The journey of self-discovery knows no age limit; it is a perpetual odyssey fueled by curiosity and courage. So, to every woman who feels the weight of time bearing down, remember this: The beauty of life lies not in its chronology, but in the ceaseless capacity for renewal and reinvention. It's never too late to script a new chapter of your story!

Once I was feeling the weight of this same pressure. What do I do about it? I climbed Mt. Fuji!

I was living in Japan at the time, where Mt. Fuji is located. I was not in the mood to sit still any longer. I was tired of being told "sorry, it's too late." So instead of accepting "no," I said "yes!" I found some friends and we climbed together. I'd never climbed a mountain before.

Climbing Mount Fuji is indeed a transformative odyssey, where every step is physically painful but emotionally awe-inspiring. The journey unfolds through a tapestry of rugged landscapes, where trails wind through dense forests, past cascading waterfalls, and across rugged volcanic terrain. The ascent is punctuated by moments of quiet introspection and shared camaraderie, as climbers from all corners of the globe unite in pursuit of a common goal.

Our climb began in the middle of the night, so we needed a flashlight and a headlamp to see the trail, as well as oxygen to help with breathing. It was like trudging through tar, only the tar had dangerous drop off points and we couldn't get a good deep breath because of the altitude. It was scary and exhausting and I kept asking myself, "What on earth was I thinking?" While I had fleeting thoughts of regret, I pushed on because that's what women do. We push on and through the boundaries and barriers in front of us. That's what I kept telling myself at least.

Step after step, as the night sky gave way to the soft glow of dawn, we reached the summit where the ethereal beauty of the sunrise cast a spell of wonder upon everyone. At the summit, where earth meets sky, we stood in silent reverence, gazing out at the world below, our spirits lifted by the boundless expanse of possibility that stretched before us. Climbing Mount Fuji was not just a physical feat, but a soul-stirring journey that left an indelible imprint on my heart and mind.

That day on the mountain, I pushed my boundaries further than ever before. The ascent of Mount Fuji wasn't just a physical conquest; it was a declaration of personal freedom and defiance against societal constraints. As a woman, the weight of societal expectations may have often felt like a heavy cloak, stifling the urge to break free and embrace the unknown. Perhaps for years, the pressure to conform to the role of a "good girl" lingers, casting shadows over dreams and desires. And now, in the years beyond 50, that pressure may loom larger than ever.

But atop Mount Fuji, amidst the crisp air and panoramic view, I made a solemn vow to break free from those chains of expectation. It's time for you too! So cast aside the shackles of conformity and embrace the spirit of adventure with open arms. The mountain taught me that life's greatest joys lie in the uncharted territories beyond our comfort zones. To every woman who has ever felt the tug of societal norms holding her back, I say this: It's time to reclaim your narrative, to seek out adventure, and to boldly say "yes" to the call of the unknown.

What is your Mt. Fuji? You don't have to go to Japan and climb a volcano. You can find your personal Mt Fuji right in your own backyard. It might be learning a new skill, starting a passion project, or embarking on a journey of self-discovery. Your Mount Fuji is whatever challenges you to grow, whatever ignites your spirit with excitement and possibility. So, take a leap of faith, step outside of your comfort zone, and pursue that dream that has been whispering to your soul. Whether it's conquering a fear, pursuing a long-held aspiration, or simply embracing the joy of spontaneity, your Mt. Fuji awaits. Embrace the journey, savor the moments of triumph, and let the spirit of adventure guide you to new heights.

Climb with me!

CHAPTER 25

Empower the Women Around You

When we empower others, we create a ripple effect of empowerment.

Standing at the base camp of Mount Everest is an experience that transcends words. Surrounded by towering peaks and vast glaciers, it's a convergence of awe-inspiring natural beauty and a profound sense of human achievement. You can't help but feel humbled not only by the mountain's grandeur, but also by the diverse community of climbers and guides preparing for the final ascent.

How do I know this? I was there!

Getting to base camp was more than I bargained for. Admittedly, I asked myself if it had been a good choice to climb. But when I arrived, I discovered a profound truth that's never left me. Before I share that truth with you, let me answer your first question: What was I doing there in the first place? Believe me, I was wondering about that myself on the way up.

The climb to the base camp of Mount Everest was a test of both my physical and mental endurance. I trained for months beforehand, getting in better shape. But as I navigated treacherous terrain, extreme altitudes, and unpredictable weather conditions, I realized no training regime could have really prepared me for this. It was probably the hardest thing I'd ever done.

I said "I" but I didn't go alone. I was joined by a few hometown friends. Together we worked our way through dense forests and picturesque villages, offering glimpses of the towering peaks that lay ahead.

As we ascended higher into the Himalayas, the landscape became increasingly rugged. One of the most daunting challenges of the climb was the altitude. As we gained elevation, the air became thinner, making each step feel like a Herculean effort. Base camp sits at nearly 18,000 ft, which was about three times the elevation of the beautiful Blue Ridge Mountains I was much more familiar with. I struggled to breath; it was a little scary at times. Every breath you take reminds you where you are!

But amidst my many deep breaths, there was also beauty and wonder to be found. The Himalayas are home to some of the most breathtaking scenery on Earth, with sweeping vistas of snow-capped peaks, deep valleys, and glittering glaciers stretching out as far as the eye can see. And as we approached the base camp of Mount Everest, it was probably the most awe-inspiring scene I'd ever seen. For my friends and me, it was also a real sense of accomplishment.

There's a palpable sense of camaraderie at base camp, as you share stories, laughter, and the occasional nervous glance with your fellow adventurers. Each person here is united by a common goal – to conquer the mighty Everest – yet each journey is deeply personal and unique. The atmosphere is one of anticipation and preparation. Small huts dot the landscape, forming a temporary village that serves as a sanctuary for weary travelers. The sound of chatter and activity fills the air as climbers gear up, check their equipment, and make final preparations for the arduous journey ahead.

However, I didn't go any further up the mountain. Getting to base camp was my goal, and I made it. My goal was much higher than base camp though, not literally but figuratively, which brings me to why I climbed in the first place.

I was motivated to climb to base camp by others, friends and colleagues, who did so to inspire other women around the world. We climbed to raise awareness and money for water accessibility to those parts of the world where clean water is hard to find. We also climbed to show other women that they can empower themselves. That's the truth that I discovered when I reached base camp. And wow did it change my world!

While my climb was difficult, women around the world must sometimes travel many miles in some pretty scary situations just to obtain water for their families. Sometimes this takes their entire day, every day, and that water is not even safe to drink, causing concern about water-borne illnesses and child mortality. So, while I was thrilled to have made the climb, I was also reminded that for many women, life is a daily climb.

When I looked up at the stars the night before we descended, which were the brightest stars I'd ever seen, it hit me: My job, the reason I was placed on this planet, was to empower women.

The profound truth that lies at the heart of personal empowerment for women is that we often overlook one of the most potent sources of strength – the act of empowering others. As women, we often find ourselves seeking empowerment in various forms – be it in our careers, relationships, or personal growth. Yet, in our quest for empowerment, we forget to empower each other.

This is what empowerment truly means. Empowerment is not merely about gaining control or authority; it is about fostering a sense of agency, confidence, and self-worth. When we empower ourselves, we tap into our inner reservoirs of strength and resilience, allowing us to navigate life's challenges with grace. And when we empower others, we create a ripple effect of empowerment that reverberates through our communities and beyond. Whether through mentorship, encouragement, or simply lending a listening ear, we have the power to profoundly impact the lives of women around us.

Empowerment is what gives women the drive to change the world! When women empower other women, it allows us to

- Celebrate each other's achievements!
- Defy norms that seek to divide us!
- Create a culture of abundance and wealth!
- Find our unique voice!
- Create spaces of empathy and healing!

What does this mean for you? When you're feeling like you have no power over your life, over your relationships, your work, even in your marriage or family, it's time to shift your focus outward. Look beyond your own struggles and challenges and seek out other women who are in need of empowerment. Climb not just for yourself but for them too! It's a transformative act of solidarity and compassion. And it's not as daunting as it may seem. There are women next door and women on the other side of the world who need help, support, and encouragement.

Whether it's offering a listening ear to a friend going through a tough time, mentoring a colleague who is struggling in their career, or volunteering your time to support women's empowerment initiatives globally, there are countless ways to make a meaningful difference in the lives of others. By lifting each other up and standing together in solidarity, we not only empower ourselves but also create a ripple effect of positive change that reverberates far beyond our immediate circles.

Will you join me?

CHAPTER 26

Remain Open to Change

When the familiar paths are blocked, it offers a unique opportunity to rediscover.

Sometimes change happens when you least expect it, and when you least want it.

My friend Nancy was in her early forties when she faced a profound life crisis. She had recently married the love of her life, and they were filled with ambitious plans for the future. Together, they dreamed of starting a family and making a significant impact on the world. Her husband, Jim, was a rising star in politics, serving as the Secretary of State of Montana and leading in a competitive three-way race for Governor. The world was their oyster, as they say.

Tragically, everything changed when the small plane Jim was aboard crashed. At that moment, Nancy's world shattered alongside the wreckage. They had been married for only eight months. Not only did she endure the heartbreak of losing her beloved husband, but she also faced the painful erosion of their shared dreams and even her hopes of becoming a mother. It was a sudden and traumatic change of events.

Nancy, a woman profoundly grounded in her faith, found herself grappling with anger towards God during this dark period of her life. Her faith, which had once been a cornerstone of her identity, felt as though it was hanging by a thread. She recalls feeling hollow, engulfed in anger and a profound sense of betrayal. During her moments of despair, she managed to whisper a small, barely audible prayer through clenched teeth: "I trust." Yet, deep down, she felt as though she had surrendered all hope. For the next six to seven months, she endured what she describes as "bone-ripping pain," a relentless agony that seemed to consume her very being.

Until one day she received an unexpected phone call that brought a glimmer of light. Her phone rang, and she answered it to hear a male voice on the other end. The caller introduced himself, saying, "Mrs. Waltermire, I've been praying for you ever since Jim died. I'd like to meet with you today for tea." At that moment, Nancy's thoughts wavered between despair and indifference—tea or arsenic, it hardly mattered to her. But in a quiet, desperate plea, she whispered to God, "Take my pain and make something beautiful out of it for your kingdom." The constant weight of her pain had worn her down, and she was reaching a point where something had to give. As she spoke to Charlie, the man on the phone, a subtle but profound realization dawned on her: This was a message from God.

When they met, Charlie's first words to her were, "God would have you know that He loves you very much." These simple words, spoken with sincere empathy, began to soften the hard edges of her grief, hinting at a new path forward out of the depths of her despair. Gradually she came out of the dark place she was in, and she started to engage and participate in life again.

"When you have a relationship with your Creator," she told me, "He'll direct your paths. He'll create the circumstances under which your potential is realized.

He came and pulled me out of it. He placed potential in each of us. Now I am so thankful for the beautiful day and this life."

Indeed, sometimes life demands new energy. Today my friend Nancy looks for opportunities to help other women not feel alone. "We're much weaker when we're isolated. We're stronger together," she says.

For many women, all of us really, life often presents unexpected challenges and unwanted situations that can feel overwhelming and disheartening. It's precisely during these turbulent times that finding new energy becomes crucial. When the familiar paths are blocked and the planned journeys disrupted, it offers a unique opportunity to rediscover your strengths and perhaps redefine your goals. Embracing these moments can lead to unexplored opportunities and new beginnings. We can transform adversity into a catalyst for growth and renewal.

It's important to remain open to change and actively seek out the silver linings, allowing them to energize and inspire your next steps forward. It's also important that we women stick close to each other. That's what a Supernova does. She releases life giving elements to those that come behind and in doing so, she can give birth to new stars. Nancy, not being one to sit still for long, says, "If we don't get involved in the game, we abdicate the playing field to whoever else is ready to play. If capable, aware women don't take hold of the opportunity, we are part of the problem."

It's difficult to find new energy after such a devastating loss. But Nancy was able to realize that she actually had a passion and a responsibility to use her experience and wisdom and network to make a difference in the world. We have so many women in our tribe that are going through transitions. Some are tragic, others not so much but still life-altering. Yet having a tribe or a group to count on for support will see you through.

Let's find new energy, together.

CHAPTER 27

It's Time to Fly Away!

As we grow older, it's easy to fall into comfortable patterns and not stray from what we know.

I met Cole on a cool but sunny morning, with a slight breeze ruffling the leaves. It was a perfect day to learn to fly.

Cole was the flight instructor who drew the lucky number and got to take me up on my first flight ever, where I was in the pilot's seat! This brave, calm, and knowledgeable young man covered all the checklists with me. (There are SO many!). He explained how to maneuver the plane on the ground and in the air, how to switch from one gas tank to another to keep the flow of fuel even, how to speed up and slow down, and how to increase and decrease elevation. He showed me how all the instruments on the panel worked, how to talk to the tower, check the weather, and establish my location.

My head was SO full of information that it was spinning. All I could think was, "I really don't want this guy to die on my watch!"

Everything was counter-intuitive. My body wanted to drive a car, but flying was so different, and I felt like I had control of nothing! I told Cole I didn't want to look like I was driving drunk down the runway. Then he said to go ahead and start climbing. I pulled back on the yoke slowly. "Keep the dash in line with the horizon," he said.

He never appeared anxious or even broke a sweat! I don't know if I would have trusted myself not to kill him, but he seemed confident and said, "We are not going to do anything dangerous." Then I asked, just to calm down, "I can't do anything wrong that you can't fix, right?" And he said, "That's right." My heart calmed down a bit. I took a deep breath and rested in the fact that even though my head was swimming in information overload, and my body felt completely like a fish out of water, Cole was calm, and there was nothing I could do that would completely mess things up. What I was feeling was normal.

And I was flying! Just like that. Terrified and thrilled all at the same time. My next big adventure.

But why?

What would make me want to do something so scary and so uncomfortable? The better question is, "Why not?"

Flying is a great new way to use and stretch my brain and my physical coordination, to learn something new. It takes focus and commitment, raises my self-confidence, and makes my life even more exciting than it already is.

As we grow older, it's easy to fall into comfortable patterns and not stray too far from what we know, avoiding big risks. But we need to remember that what stops growing begins to die. We become less interesting, less curious, and less interested in life. Sure, it's good to have a routine, but it's also healthy to choose adventures and learn new things.

New experiences challenge us to step out of our comfort zones, which is essential for personal growth. The thrill of trying something new invigorates us and helps us stay mentally sharp and physically active. Whether it's flying a plane, learning a new language, taking up a new hobby, or even traveling to a new place, these adventures bring excitement and a fresh perspective to our lives.

When you have a sense of purpose and growth and a curious mind, you live longer and are healthier, mentally and physically.

I want my 20 grandchildren to be able to look at each other, shake their heads in amazement, and say, "What's grandma up to now?" They may laugh, but as they grow, they will know that life is a fabulous adventure and that they, too, can do and accomplish anything they choose. And the world will be a happier place because of it.

Taking on new challenges also sets a powerful example for those around us. It shows that it's never too late to learn, to grow, and to embrace life fully. By continuously seeking out new adventures, we inspire others to do the same, fostering a culture of lifelong learning and exploration.

What's YOUR next adventure going to be? Go for it!

Remember, life's greatest adventures often come when we step beyond our fears and embrace the unknown. So take that leap, pursue that dream, and let the journey unfold.

You might be surprised at just how far you can go!

Printed in the USA
CPSIA information can be obtained
at www.ICGtesting.com
LVHW040247220824
788890LV00005B/107

9 781963 701999